Richard Warren · Alan Men

D0986018

Handbook of
Psoriasis and
Psoriatic Arthritis

Richard Warren, MBChB, FRCP, PhD
The University of Manchester
Salford Royal Foundation Hospital
Manchester, UK

Alan Menter, MD
Division of Dermatology
Baylor University Medical Center
Dallas, Texas, USA

Handbook of Psoriasis and Psoriatic Arthritis

△ Adis

Editors

Richard Warren, MBChB, FRCP, PhD
The University of Manchester
Salford Royal Foundation Hospital
Manchester, UK

Alan Menter, MD
Division of Dermatology
Baylor University Medical Center
Dallas, Texas, USA

Contributors

Matthias Augustin, MD
Laura Coates, MD, PhD
Musaab Elmamoun, MBBS, MRCP
Paul Emery, MD, FRCP
Oliver Fitzgerald, MD, FRCP, FRCPI
Kenneth B Gordon, MD
Rebecca I Hartman, MD, MPH
Alexa B Kimball, MD, MPH
Marc Alexander Radtke, MD
Eric Ruderman, MD
Laura Savage, MD
Zenas Yiu, MBChB, MRCP

ISBN 978-3-319-18226-1   ISBN 978-3-319-18227-8 (eBook)
DOI 10.1007/978-3-319-18227-8
Springer Cham Heidelberg New York Dordrecht London

Printed on acid-free paper

Adis is a brand of Springer
Springer is part of Springer Science+Business Media (www.springer.com)

Project editors: Laura Hajba

Contents

5 Treatment of psoriasis   43

Matthias Augustin and Marc Alexander Radtke

6 Treatment of psoriatic arthritis   85

Musaab Elmamoun and Oliver Fitzgerald

Matthias Augustin and Marc Alexander Radtke

Editor biographies

Richard Warren, MBChB, MRCP, PhD, is a Clinical Senior Lecturer and Honorary Consultant Dermatologist. He graduated from Liverpool University with a first class honours degree in Pharmacology and gained his Medical degree, with honours, one year later. He was awarded The J Hill Abram prize – highest mark in Medicine; and the Reginald Dora Goodrick prize – highest mark in Surgery. His work in Dermatology has focused on: pharmacogenetics (forming the basis of his PhD thesis), the genetic susceptibility to psoriasis and more recently biological therapies and their use in the treatment of psoriasis. For his work into the pharmacogenetics of methotrexate he has received national and international awards from the British Association of Dermatologists (BAD) and American Academy of Dermatology. He is widely published in the field of dermatology with numerous abstracts, papers and book contributions including *The Lancet, Nature Genetics,* and *The Journal of Investigative Dermatology.* He is currently the EU Editor in Chief for the journal *Dermatology and Therapy.* He has been an invited plenary speaker at major national and international dermatology meetings and is a member of The International Psoriasis Council. He currently chairs the BAD guideline group for methotrexate and is a member of the BAD biologics committee and research subcommittee. In 2012, he was the expert panel member on the National Institute for Health and Clinical Excellence guideline group for psoriasis. He co-lead one of the two workstreams involved in the recent (2013) successful funding from the Medical Research Council stratified medicine grant (value £7 million) – Psoriasis Optimisation of Relevant Therapies (PSORT). He co-established a clinic for patients with severe psoriasis and psoriatic arthritis in 2010 with Dr Hector Chinoy, which has received wide acclaim and is used as a national exemplar.

Alan Menter, MD, was born in England and is a graduate of the Medical School of the University of Witwatersrand, South Africa. He completed his dermatology residency at Pretoria General Hospital at the University of Pretoria, also in South Africa, and two fellowships in London at Guy's

Hospital and St John's Hospital for Diseases of the Skin. A fellowship with the University of Texas Southwestern Medical Center in Dallas brought Menter to the United States. Since then, he has held several positions within the UT and Baylor University Dallas systems. In 1992, he was appointed Chairman of the Division of Dermatology at Baylor University Medical Center and still holds that position. In 2007, he was appointed Director of the Baylor Research Center and in 2010, Program Director of the newly formed Dermatology Residency Program at Baylor University Medical Center.

Dr Menter has a long-held interest in psoriasis and psoriatic disease research. In 1994, he co-authored the first gene discovery for psoriasis, published in *Science* in 1994. His research on psoriasis has examined everything from ultraviolet phototherapy and biologic therapy to the mapping of genetic patterns to predict if a person is at risk of developing psoriasis pharmacogenomics. In August 2004, Dr Menter helped found the International Psoriasis Council to raise international awareness of psoriasis as a serious autoimmune disease that can significantly impact quality of life. His clinical practice includes more than 1600 patients on systemic and biologic therapy.

Dr Menter held the position of clinical director of the National Psoriasis Foundation Gene Bank from 1996 to 2002. His resume lists some 300+ articles, four books and 19 book chapters. He serves as a member of the editorial board for several medical journals, including the *Journal of Clinical Dermatology* and *Clinical and Experimental Dermatology*. He is chair of research for Dermatology at Baylor Research Institute, as well as clinical professor of dermatology at the University of Texas Southwestern Medical School in Dallas and professor at Texas A&M Health Science Center, College of Medicine. Dr Menter has been listed in the Best Doctors in America since 1994 and Who's Who in Medicine and Healthcare since 1996. He also represented the South African National Rugby team, the Springboks, in 1968. In 2013, Dr Menter received the Lifetime Achievement Award from the National Psoriasis Foundation. In March 2015, he received the Dermatology Foundation annual Clark W. Finnerud award at the American Academy of Dermatology 2015 meeting in San Francisco.

Abbreviations

ACR20	American College of Rheumatology 20 response rate
AS	Ankylosing spondylitis
ASAS	Assessment of Spondyloarthritis International Society
CASPAR	Classification of Criteria for Psoriatic Arthritis
CCP	Cyclic citrullinated peptides
CRP	C-reactive protein
DIP	Distal interphalangeal
DISH	Diffuse idiopathic skeletal hyperostosis
ESR	Erythocyte sedimentation rate
GRAPPA	Group for the Assessment of Psoriasis and Psoriatic Arthritis
GWAS	Genome-wide association studies
HIV	Human immunodeficiency virus
HLA	Human leukocyte antigen
IBD	Inflammatory bowel disease
IL	Interleukin
LEI	Leeds Enthesitis Index
MEI	Mander Enthesitis Index
MRI	Magnetic resonance imaging
mSASS	The modified Stoke Ankylosing Spondylitis Spinal Score
NAPSI	Nail Psoriasis Severity Index
OA	Osteoarthritis
OMERACT	Outcomes Measures in Rheumatology
PsA	Psoriatic arthritis
PsARC	Psoriatic Arthritis Response Criteria
RA	Rheumatoid arthritis
RANKL	Nuclear factor kappa-B ligand
RF	Rheumatoid factor
SpA	Spondyloarthritis
TNF	Tumor necrosis factor
VA	Veterans Affairs

Chapter 1

Introduction

Zenas Yiu, Richard Warren, and Alan Menter

The aim of this handbook is to provide the reader with an overview of key topics on psoriasis and psoriatic arthritis (PsA), ranging from the etiology, immunopathogenesis, and clinical presentation to quality of life measures, diagnosis, and treatment options. The book is targeted at those who have an interest in skin disease and joint disease such as dermatologists, rheumatologists, primary care physicians, and other healthcare providers who may encounter these conditions. The format is one of a concise, accessible, and evidence-based text, which has an emphasis on clinically relevant practice points.

Disease overview and epidemiology

Psoriasis is a chronic cutaneous inflammatory disease manifesting as erythematous, raised, well-demarcated plaques with adherent scales. Robert Willian (1757–1812) was the first physician to accurately describe and classify psoriasis, and his description will be familiar to many medical students and physicians looking after psoriasis patients today: "…(Cutaneous psoriasis) retain a circular or oval form, and are covered with dry scales, and surrounded by a red border. Scales accumulate on them, so as to form a thick crust…". The extent of skin involvement in psoriasis can vary from a few sparse areas of erythema on the elbows to thick plaque involvement of multiple highly visible sites such as the hands and the scalp, while severe unstable disease can involve the whole

© Springer International Publishing Switzerland 2016   1
R. Warren and A. Menter (eds.), *Handbook of Psoriasis
and Psoriatic Arthritis*, DOI 10.1007/978-3-319-18227-8_1

body. A national cross-sectional survey in the United States estimates the prevalence of psoriasis to be approximately 2% [1], while the global prevalence of psoriasis in adults ranges from 0.91% (United States) to 8.5% (Norway) [2]. The global incidence of psoriasis also varies from 78.9/100,000 person-years (United States) to 230/100,000 person-years (Italy). There is a discrepancy in the frequency of psoriasis according to geographical region, with an increasing frequency of disease the further the country is from the equator. There is also a bimodal distribution of the incidence of psoriasis with age, with peaks between the ages of 20–29 and the ages of 50–59. Psoriasis has equal gender preponderance.

PsA is a sero-negative inflammatory polyarthropathy, with typical presentations including dactylitis (swelling of an entire digit) and enthesitis (tendon insertion inflammation). Moll and Wright (1973) first described five subgroups of PsA in their diagnostic criteria: asymmetrical oligoarthritis, polyarthritis, spondylitis, arthritis mutilans, and distal interphalangeal joint involvement only. Although these were useful descriptions of the clinical manifestations of PsA, diagnostic criteria have been superseded by validated scoring systems (eg, CASPAR classification), which although designed for classifying the disease have been found to be both highly sensitive and specific when making the diagnosis of PsA. Prior to the formation of these scores, epidemiological studies on PsA were difficult to interpret. Prevalence of PsA in the general population ranges from 0.02% to 0.4%, with the global incidence at approximately 6.4 cases per 100,000 [3]. The prevalence of psoriasis patients with PsA is between 7 and 24% [4], with over 86% of patients with PsA presenting with psoriasis prior to the onset of PsA by around 15 years [5]. The age of onset of PsA is in the range of 30–55 years, and as with psoriasis it also has an equal sex distribution, although men are more likely to develop axial PsA and radiographic joint damage [6]. It is uncertain whether any clinical characteristics of the psoriasis patients can accurately predict future development of PsA, although some studies suggest the occurrence of nail dystrophy [7,8] and trauma [9] as probable predictors. There is a current research emphasis on identifying genetic and epidemiological risk factors that predispose and potentially lead to the development of PsA. This would allow for the identification of psoriasis patients at a high risk of developing PsA and thus ensure early intervention, which has been shown to improve clinical outcome [10].

Prognosis, morbidity, and mortality

The severity of psoriasis can fluctuate, with factors such as genetic heritage, physiological and psychogenic stress, smoking, and hormonal changes playing a role in the exacerbation of the disease. Despite recent advances in the knowledge of the immunopathogenesis and increasing therapeutic options for psoriasis, little is known about the natural history of the disease [11]. It is thought that environmental risk factors may predispose a person to the development of psoriasis, but to date the mechanism by which this may happen has not been defined. PsA can follow an aggressive course, with 20% of patients developing a destructive arthropathy, and 67% of patients in clinics found to have evidence of joint erosion [12]. However, a recent longitudinal study has found that patients with psoriasis, and not PsA, have a severity-dependent increased mortality risk [13].

People with psoriasis suffer from a reduced quality of life leading to significant loss of productivity, with the extent of this effect comparable to patients with other significant illnesses such as cancer, diabetes, and depression [14]. Psoriasis patients often have a fear of relapse and stigmatization, resulting in high levels of psychological distress [15,16]. People suffering from both psoriasis and PsA have an even lower quality of life than psoriasis alone [17].

Associated comorbidities

Inflammatory bowel disease is closely associated with psoriasis, with Crohn's disease patients having five times the risk of developing psoriasis as compared with a control population. Psoriasis is also associated with comorbidities including metabolic syndrome, type 2 diabetes mellitus, depression, and non-alcoholic fatty liver disease. Severe psoriasis is associated with an increased cardiovascular disease risk, with increased risk of mortality due to myocardial infarction and stroke [18]. Whether the association is causal, with systemic inflammation in psoriasis affecting formation of atherosclerotic plaques and rupture, or due to increased underlying traditional cardiovascular risk factors, such as smoking, excess alcohol intake, and the other comorbidities listed above, is under hot debate. What is clear, however, is that holistic management of the lifestyle risk factors and a heightened vigilance for the associated comorbidities is of paramount importance in the treatment of psoriasis.

Therapeutics

For many years treatment with methotrexate was the only effective option for treating both psoriasis and PsA, with other therapies, such as leflunomide and cyclosporine, being joint- or skin-specific in terms of efficacy. The advent of biologic therapies, specifically the tumor necrosis factor-α antagonists (anti-TNFs) such as infliximab, etanercept and adalimumab, has transformed the level of care for both conditions. Other novel anti-TNFs, certolizumab and golimumab, are also in clinical use for the treatment of PsA, and also show efficacy for the treatment of psoriasis. Further agents have been developed with clinical utility in both conditions. Ustekinumab, an interleukin (IL)-12/23 inhibitor, has been licensed for the treatment of psoriasis for more than five years and affords an excellent therapeutic response. Recent clinical trial data demonstrate that it is also efficacious for the treatment of PsA, albeit at a lower level than anti-TNFs. The IL-17 antagonists secukinumab, ixekizumab, and brodalumab have shown very high levels of efficacy for psoriasis in clinical trials through targeted blockade of the T-helper cell 17 pathway, and emerging data are also showing significant promise in the treatment of PsA. Besides the biologic therapies, novel small molecule therapies have been developed, which deliver ease of monitoring and administration. Apremilast, orally dosed phosphodiesterase 4 inhibitor, has shown impressive efficacy and a favorable safety profile in patients with PsA. It has also proven to be effective in around a third of patients with psoriasis. Apremilast is approved in the USA for PsA without the need for screening and regular laboratory monitoring, and may prove a good option in those with comorbidities.

In summary, this book will give an update on our current and evolving understanding of the etiology of psoriasis and PsA and as a consequence the rapidly expanding therapeutic armamentarium being used to treat these potentially life-ruining conditions.

References

1 Stern RS, Nijsten T, Feldman SR, Margolis DJ, Rolstad T. Psoriasis is common, carries a substantial burden even when not extensive, and is associated with widespread treatment dissatisfaction. *J Investig Dermatol Symp Proc*. 2004;9:136-139.

2 Parisi R, Symmons DP, Griffiths CE, et al. Global epidemiology of psoriasis: a systematic review of incidence and prevalence. *J Invest Dermatol*. 2013;133:377-385.

3 Alamanos Y, Voulgari PV, Drosos AA. Incidence and prevalence of psoriatic arthritis: a systematic review. *J Rheumatol*. 2008;35:1354-1358.

4 Prey S, Paul C, Bronsard V, et al. Assessment of risk of psoriatic arthritis in patients with plaque psoriasis: a systematic review of the literature. *J Eur Acad Dermatol Venereol*. 2010;24:31-35.

5 Armstrong AW, Schupp C, Bebo B. Psoriasis comorbidities: results from the National Psoriasis Foundation surveys 2003 to 2011. *Dermatology*. 2012;225:121-126.

6 Eder L, Thavaneswaran A, Chandran V, Gladman DD. Gender difference in disease expression, radiographic damage and disability among patients with psoriatic arthritis. *Ann Rheum Dis*. 2013;72:578-582.

7 Wilson FC, Icen M, Crowson CS, McEvoy MT, Gabriel SE, Kremers HM. Incidence and clinical predictors of psoriatic arthritis in patients with psoriasis: a population-based study. *Arthritis Rheum*. 2009;61:233-239.

8 Langenbruch A, Radtke MA, Krensel M, Jacobi A, Reich K, Augustin M. Nail involvement as a predictor of concomitant psoriatic arthritis in patients with psoriasis. *Br J Dermatol*. 2014;171:1123-1128.

9 Pattison E, Harrison BJ, Griffiths CE, Silman AJ, Bruce IN. Environmental risk factors for the development of psoriatic arthritis: results from a case-control study. *Ann Rheum Dis*. 2008;67:672-676.

10 Theander E, Husmark T, Alenius GM. Early psoriatic arthritis: short symptom duration, male gender and preserved physical functioning at presentation predict favourable outcome at 5-year follow-up. Results from the Swedish Early Psoriatic Arthritis Register (SwePsA). *Ann Rheum Dis*. 2014;73:407-413.

11 Farber EM, Nall ML. The natural history of psoriasis in 5,600 patients. *Dermatologica*. 1974;148:1-18.

12 Gladman DD, Antoni C, Mease P, Clegg DO, Nash P. Psoriatic arthritis: epidemiology, clinical features, course, and outcome. *Ann Rheum Dis*. 2005;64:ii14-ii17.

13 Ogdie A, Haynes K, Troxel AB, et al. Risk of mortality in patients with psoriatic arthritis, rheumatoid arthritis and psoriasis: a longitudinal cohort study. *Ann Rheum Dis*. 2014;73: 149-153.

14 Rapp SR, Feldman SR, Exum ML, Fleischer AB Jr, Reboussin DM. Psoriasis causes as much disability as other major medical diseases. *J Am Acad Dermatol*. 1999;41:401-417.

15 Richards HL, Fortune DG, Griffiths CE, Main CJ. The contribution of perceptions of stigmatisation to disability in patients with psoriasis. *J Psychosom Res*. 2001;50:11-15.

16 Fortune DG, Richards HL, Griffiths CE. Psychologic factors in psoriasis: consequences, mechanisms, and interventions. *Dermatol Clin*. 2005;23:681-694.

17 Rosen CF, Mussani F, Chandran V, Eder L, Thavaneswaran A, Gladman DD. Patients with psoriatic arthritis have worse quality of life than those with psoriasis alone. *Rheumatology (Oxford)*. 2012;51:571-576.

18 Samarasekera EJ, Neilson JM, Warren RB, Parnham J, Smith CH. Incidence of cardiovascular disease in individuals with psoriasis: a systematic review and meta-analysis. *J Invest Dermatol*. 2013;133:2340-2346.

Chapter 2

Pathogenesis of psoriasis and psoriatic arthritis

Laura Coates, Laura Savage, and Paul Emery

Pathophysiology of psoriasis

The pathophysiology of psoriasis is multifaceted and dynamic, involving a complex interplay between constitutive cells of the skin and the innate and adaptive immune systems. Until the early 1980s, psoriasis was considered to be primarily a disease of epidermal keratinocyte proliferation, with the cutaneous inflammatory infiltrate a secondary consequence [1]. However, the effective use of therapies designed to inhibit T-cell activation, such as cyclosporine [2] in the late 1970s, and interleukin (IL)-2 toxin [3] and alefacept [4,5] (lymphocyte function-associated antigen3-Ig) and IL-17A [6] more latterly, has led to a paradigm shift in psoriasis pathogenesis to an immune cell-mediated inflammatory etiology.

Over the past decade, evidence from mouse models and translational research strongly indicates that psoriatic plaques result from both a primary defect in keratinocytes and an inappropriate innate and adaptive immune response mediated mainly by resident and infiltrating T cells [7–10]. Psoriatic skin lesions are highly infiltrated most notably with $CD3^+$ T lymphocytes, $CD4^+$ T helper cells and $CD11c^+$ myeloid dendritic cells within the dermis [11,12], and CD8+ T cells and neutrophils in the epidermis [13]. Complex interactions between these T cells,

© Springer International Publishing Switzerland 2016
R. Warren and A. Menter (eds.), *Handbook of Psoriasis and Psoriatic Arthritis*, DOI 10.1007/978-3-319-18227-8_2

dendritic cells, keratinocytes, neutrophils and the proinflammatory cytokines produced by these cells – including tumour necrosis factor alpha (TNF-α), interferon-gamma (IFN-γ), IL-17, IL-22, IL-23, IL-12 and IL-1β – contribute to the initiation and perpetuation of cutaneous inflammation characteristic of psoriasis [14,15].

Etiology

Population studies clearly signify a genetic association in psoriasis, with the incidence being greater amongst first-degree and second-degree relatives of patients than among the general population [16,17]. Genetic linkage and subsequent genome wide association studies (GWAS) have confirmed associations with numerous polymorphisms within genes involved in: (i) immune regulation such as IL-23 signalling (IL-23A, IL-12B and IL-23R) [18–21] and nuclear factor (NF)-κB signalling (*REL, TNIP1, TRAF31P2, TNFAIP3, KFKBIA, FBXL19,* and *CARD14*) [18,19,22,23]; (ii) barrier function (late cornified envelope (LCE) proteins 3B and 3C) [18]; and (iii) epidermal microbial defence (DEFB4) [24]. These analyses add confirmation to the definition of psoriasis as an immune cell-mediated disease of defective keratinocytes [25], although the precise functional effects of these associated single nucleotide polymorphisms remain to be determined.

The locus with the largest effect identified to date in genetic studies of psoriasis is PSORS1, a major histocompatibility complex (MHC) class I region on chromosome 6p21 [26]. Within PSORS1, the human leukocyte antigen (HLA)-Cw06 allele is pinpointed as the risk variant that confers the strongest susceptibility to psoriasis [27]. However, only 60–65% of patients with psoriasis carry the *HLA-Cw06* gene, compared with 15% of individuals without psoriasis [28]. Furthermore, a low penetrance of approximately 10% points towards other genetic and environmental factors being involved [29].

In individuals with a genetic predisposition, external stimuli such as trauma (Koebner phenomenon), infections, stress, drugs, and alcohol can all trigger an initial episode of psoriasis through activation of the innate immune system. A cascade of immunological events then ensues, leading to a persistent inflammatory state within the skin:

- Following epidermal damage, 'stressed' keratinocytes release both LL-37 (cathelicidin) antimicrobial peptide and host DNA/RNA, which together activate plasmacytoid dendritic cells to produce large quantities of interferon (IFN)-alpha [9,30,31].
- IFN-alpha induces the maturation of myeloid (dermal) dendritic cells, which in turn produce cytokines including IL-23 and IL-12 [8].
- IL-23 and IL-12 stimulate the attraction, activation and differentiation of T cells within skin draining lymph nodes, thereby bridging the gap between the innate and adaptive immune systems [32]. Subsequent T-cell expansion and migration into the epidermis (through expression of α1β1 integrin) results in characteristic epidermal remodeling [10].
- Differentiated psoriatic T cells are of two distinctly polarised types [33,34]: IFN-gamma secreting T helper 1 (Th1) cells [35] and Th17 cells, which when influenced by IL-23 [35–37] produce IL-17 and IL-22 [39–41].
- IFN-gamma enhances expression of MHC class I on keratinocytes, which may promote presentation of putative autoantigens to intra-epidermal T cells. In turn, this may lead to further activation of pathogenic autoimmune T cells [42].
- IL-17 and IL-22 are key mediators linking the adaptive immune response and epithelial dysregulation in psoriasis [43,44]:
  - IL-22 causes keratinocyte hyperproliferation (seen histologically as acanthosis). This is enhanced by IFN-alpha which up-regulates IL-22 receptor expression on keratinocytes [45]. IL-22 therefore provides an interface between immune activation and epidermal acanthosis [45,46].
  - Both IL-17 and IL-22 increase production of LL-37 [47–49] leading to sustained production of IFN-alpha and unregulated activation of myeloid dendritic cells, thus fuelling the continued activation of the immune system through a positive feedback loop [50].

In addition to the established role of conventional T cells in the pathogenesis of psoriasis, increasing interest surrounds innate γδT cells resident within the dermis. γδT cells constitutively express the IL-23 receptor (IL-23R), and in the presence of IL-23, rapidly produce copious IL-17, thus amplifying Th17 responses [51–53]. Accumulations of γδT cells have been found in psoriatic plaques [52], as have Vγ9Vδ2 T cells (a novel proinflammatory subset that seems to mediate an immediate tissue response upon koebnerization) [54], suggesting these innate cells may play some role in psoriasis pathogenesis.

Pathophysiology of psoriatic arthritis

Psoriatic arthritis (PsA) was not recognized as a disease separate from RA until the 1950s, but since then our understanding of where PsA fits within a spectrum of spondyloarthritides alongside cutaneous psoriasis has clarified considerably. As in psoriasis, PsA seems to be associated with changes in both the innate immune system and also in the adaptive immune system with the involvement of T cells.

Etiology

Genetic factors

As with many other inflammatory arthritides, PsA was recognized to be highly heritable from early family studies. Interestingly the heritability of PsA (recurrence risk or γS estimated at 27 [55]) seems to be much greater than that of psoriasis (γS between 4 and 11) [56]. A study in Iceland confirmed the significantly increased risk ratios for development of PsA in first- to fourth-degree relatives of those with PsA (39, 12, 3.6, and 2.3, respectively, p<0.0001 [17]. On review of GWAS studies, it is clear that the majority of the genetic associations found in PsA are the same as those seen in cutaneous psoriasis, with a much smaller overlap seen with RA [57]. There are also shared genetic susceptibilities with ankylosing spondylitis (AS), including HLA-B27, IL-23R, and IL-12B [58], particularly in those with axial involvement. It has been recognized that psoriatic patients are at high risk of developing systemic co-morbidities and have an association with the metabolic syndrome. The relationship between skin disease and a co-morbid condition has recently been reviewed [59].

Environmental factors

As in cutaneous psoriasis, there is some evidence in PsA that environmental factors can trigger the disease in genetically susceptible individuals. The most reported trigger of PsA is trauma, suggested as a 'deep Koebner phenomenon' with multiple studies showing an association with acute physical trauma [60,61] or psychological trauma (eg, moving house) [62]. Infection may also be a significant trigger for PsA. Clear associations between human immunodeficiency virus (HIV) infection and psoriasis and PsA have been reported [63], and an increased prevalence of hepatitis C viral infection has been observed in patients with PsA as compared with psoriasis, RA and general population controls [64]. Despite strong links to streptococcal infections in psoriasis, particularly guttate psoriasis, there is no evidence of a relationship between such infections and the development of PsA.

Inflammatory pathways in psoriatic arthritis

Investigating inflammatory pathways in PsA is complex given the heterogeneity of the condition. PsA can result in inflammation within the synovium, entheses and spine, affecting both soft tissue and bone. Within the synovium, significant morphological changes are seen in the vasculature similar to that seen in psoriatic skin plaques and this angiogenesis has been related to functional changes in infiltrating immune cells [65]. Raised levels of proinflammatory cytokines have also been identified within the joint including p40 (a common subunit of IL-12 and IL-23), TNF-α, IL-1, IL-6, IL-8, and IL-10 with some relationships noted between cytokine levels and clinical arthritis severity [66]. There is some evidence of a relationship between synovitis and subsequent bone erosion in PsA [67] and destructive matrix metalloproteinases identified in the synovium. Severe osteolysis can also be seen in subtypes of PsA such as arthritis mutilans and there is an implication of increased osteoclastic activity in PsA. In the joint, increased receptor activator of nuclear factor kappa-B ligand (RANKL) expression is associated with activation of osteoclasts. Increased levels of osteoclast precursors have been identified in the peripheral blood of patients with PsA, which decreased after administration of anti-TNF therapies [68].

Investigation of the immunopathogenesis of enthesitis has been limited by the difficulty in obtaining appropriate material for study given the inability to biopsy entheses. Imaging studies have suggested increased vascularity at the tendon insertions as well as extracapsular inflammation seen adjacent to synovial joints and soft tissue inflammation in subcutaneous tissues in dactylitis. This led to the theory of differentiation in pathogenesis in PsA. Jevtic et al [69] first described the extensive extra-capsular inflammation seen on magnetic resonance imaging (MRI), with half of their cases showing predominantly synovial inflammation whereas other cases showed neighboring inflammation in thickened collateral ligaments and periarticular soft tissue, particularly in dactylitic joints. This research suggested that there may be heterogeneity in PsA where some patients have a predominantly synovial disease, as in RA, and some show a predominantly entheseal-driven disease, as in spondyloarthritis. After similar imaging results, McGonagle et al went on to hypothesize the primary role of enthesitis in PsA with a secondary spread of inflammation to the synovium [70].

Among the sites affected by PsA, axial involvement is perhaps the least understood. Although there are some similarities with other spondyloarthritides such as AS, different morphological patterns of spinal involvement are seen in PsA and some important genetic associations seen in AS do not apply to all patients with PsA. Radiological changes in the cervical spine occur in up to 70–75% of patients with PsA [71,72], much more common than observed in patients with sacroiliitis. Disease seen in the cervical spine is particularly interesting as it seems that two distinct pathological types occur. In 1964, Kaplan et al observed that radiological changes in the cervical spine in PsA and skin psoriasis bore a closer resemblance to AS than to RA [73]. Blau and Kaufman went on to describe two separate patterns of cervical spine disease: primarily ankylosing in nature or a rheumatoid-like form of inflammatory cervical involvement [71]. Despite the strikingly different radiological features, there seems to be no difference between the two groups in terms of clinical symptoms, however rheumatoid-like disease is associated with B39 and DR4 antigens with evidence of radiocarpal erosions [72].

References

1 Bos JD, de Rie MA, Teunissen MB, Piskin G. Psoriasis: dysregulation of innate immunity. *Br J Dermatol*. 2005;152:1098-1107.

2 Ellis CN, Gorsulowsky DC, Hamilton TA, et al. Cyclosporine improves psoriasis in a double-blind study. *JAMA*. 1986;256:3110-3116.

3 Gottlieb SL, Gilleaudeau P, Johnson R, et al. Response of psoriasis to a lymphocyte-selective toxin (DAB389IL-2) suggests a primary immune, but not keratinocyte, pathogenic basis. *Nat Med*. 1995;1:442-447.

4 Abrams JR, Kelley SL, Hayes E, et al. Blockade of T lymphocyte costimulation with cytotoxic T lymphocyte-associated antigen 4-immunoglobulin (CTLA4Ig) reverses the cellular pathology of psoriatic plaques, including the activation of keratinocytes, dendritic cells, and endothelial cells. *J Exp Med*. 2000;192:681-694.

5 Abrams JR, Lebwohl MG, Guzzo CA, et al. CTLA4Ig-mediated blockade of T-cell costimulation in patients with psoriasis vulgaris. *J Clin Invest*. 1999;103:1243-1252.

6 McInnes IB, Mease PJ, Kirkham B, et al. Secukinumab, a human anti-interleukin-17A monoclonal antibody, in patients with psoriatic arthritis (FUTURE 2): a randomised, double-blind, placebo-controlled, phase 3 trial. Lancet. 2015 [Epub ahead of print]; doi: 10.1016/S0140-6736(15)61134-5.

7 Sano S, Chan KS, Carbajal S, et al. Stat3 links activated keratinocytes and immunocytes required for development of psoriasis in a novel transgenic mouse model. *Nat Med*. 2005;11:43-49.

8 Nestle FO, Conrad C, Tun-Kyi A, et al. Plasmacytoid predendritic cells initiate psoriasis through interferon-alpha production. *J Exp Med*. 2005;202:135-143.

9 Lande R, Gregorio J, Facchinetti V, et al. Plasmacytoid dendritic cells sense self-DNA coupled with antimicrobial peptide. *Nature*. 2007;449:564-569.

10 Conrad C, Boyman O, Tonel G, et al. Alpha1beta1 integrin is crucial for accumulation of epidermal T cells and the development of psoriasis. *Nat Med*. 2007;13:836-842.

11 Lowes MA, Chamian F, Abello MV, et al. Increase in TNF-alpha and inducible nitric oxide synthase-expressing dendritic cells in psoriasis and reduction with efalizumab (anti-CD11a). *Proc Natl Acad Sci U S A*. 2005;102:19057-19062.

12 Chamian F, Lowes MA, Lin SL, et al. Alefacept reduces infiltrating T cells, activated dendritic cells, and inflammatory genes in psoriasis vulgaris. *Proc Natl Acad Sci U S A*. 2005;102:2075-2080.

13 Lowes MA, Bowcock AM, Krueger JG. Pathogenesis and therapy of psoriasis. *Nature*. 2007;445:866-873.

14 Krueger JG. Hiding under the skin: a welcome surprise in psoriasis. *Nat Med*. 2012;18:1750-1751.

15 Johnson-Huang LM, Lowes MA, Krueger JG. Putting together the psoriasis puzzle: an update on developing targeted therapies. *Dis Model Mech*. 2012;5:423-433.

16 Farber EM, Nall ML. The natural history of psoriasis in 5,600 patients. *Dermatologica*. 1974;148:1-18.

17 Karason A, Love TJ, Gudbjornsson B. A strong heritability of psoriatic arthritis over four generations–the Reykjavik Psoriatic Arthritis Study. *Rheumatology (Oxford)*. 2009;48:1424-1428.

18 Capon F, Burden AD, Trembath RC, Barker JN. Psoriasis and other complex trait dermatoses: from Loci to functional pathways. *J Invest Dermatol*. 2012;132:915-922.

19 Nair RP, Duffin KC, Helms C, et al. Genome-wide scan reveals association of psoriasis with IL-23 and NF-kappaB pathways. *Nat Genet*. 2009;41:199-204.

20 Nair RP, Ruether A, Stuart PE, et al. Polymorphisms of the IL12B and IL23R genes are associated with psoriasis. *J Investi Dermatol*. 2008;128:1653-1661.

21 Cargill M, Schrodi SJ, Chang M, et al. A large-scale genetic association study confirms IL12B and leads to the identification of IL23R as psoriasis-risk genes. *Am J Hum Genet*. 2007;80:273-290.

22 Jordan CT, Cao L, Roberson ED, et al. Rare and common variants in CARD14, encoding an epidermal regulator of NF-kappaB, in psoriasis. *Am J Hum Genet*. 2012;90:796-808.

23 Jordan CT, Cao L, Roberson ED, et al. PSORS2 is due to mutations in CARD14. *Am J Hum Genet.* 2012;90:784-795.

24 Hollox EJ, Huffmeier U, Zeeuwen PL, et al. Psoriasis is associated with increased beta-defensin genomic copy number. *Nat Genet.* 2008;40:23-25.

25 Nograles KE, Davidovici B, Krueger JG. New insights in the immunologic basis of psoriasis. *Semin Cutan Med Surg.* 2010;29:3-9.

26 Nestle FO, Kaplan DH, Barker J. Psoriasis. *N Engl J Med.* 2009;361:496-509.

27 Nair RP, Stuart PE, Nistor I, et al. Sequence and haplotype analysis supports HLA-C as the psoriasis susceptibility 1 gene. *Am J Hum Genet.* 2006;78:827-851.

28 Gudjonsson JE, Karason A, Runarsdottir EH, et al. Distinct clinical differences between HLA-Cw*0602 positive and negative psoriasis patients–an analysis of 1019 HLA-C- and HLA-B-typed patients. *J Invest Dermatol.* 2006;126):740-745.

29 Elder JT, Nair RP, Voorhees JJ. Epidemiology and the genetics of psoriasis. *J Invest Dermatol.* 1994;102:24S-27S.

30 Marrakchi S, Guigue P, Renshaw BR, et al. Interleukin-36-receptor antagonist deficiency and generalized pustular psoriasis. *N Engl J Med.* 2011;365:620-628.

31 Ganguly D, Chamilos G, Lande R, et al. Self-RNA-antimicrobial peptide complexes activate human dendritic cells through TLR7 and TLR8. *J Exp Med.* 2009;206:1983-1994.

32 Gilliet M, Cao W, Liu YJ. Plasmacytoid dendritic cells: sensing nucleic acids in viral infection and autoimmune diseases. *Nat Rev Immunol.* 2008;8:594-606.

33 Steinman L. A brief history of T(H)17, the first major revision in the T(H)1/T(H)2 hypothesis of T cell-mediated tissue damage. *Nat Med.* 2007;13:139-145.

34 Trifari S, Kaplan CD, Tran EH, Crellin NK, Spits H. Identification of a human helper T cell population that has abundant production of interleukin 22 and is distinct from T(H)-17, T(H)1 and T(H)2 cells. *Nat Immunol.* 2009;10:864-871.

35 Uyemura K, Yamamura M, Fivenson DF, Modlin RL, Nickoloff BJ. The cytokine network in lesional and lesion-free psoriatic skin is characterized by a T-helper type 1 cell-mediated response. *J Invest Dermatol.* 1993;101:701-705.

36 Lee E, Trepicchio WL, Oestreicher JL, et al. Increased expression of interleukin 23 p19 and p40 in lesional skin of patients with psoriasis vulgaris. *J Exp Med.* 2004;199:125-130.

37 Chan JR, Blumenschein W, Murphy E, et al. IL-23 stimulates epidermal hyperplasia via TNF and IL-20R2-dependent mechanisms with implications for psoriasis pathogenesis. *J Exp Med.* 2006;203:2577-2587.

38 Tonel G, Conrad C, Laggner U, et al. Cutting edge: a critical functional role for IL-23 in psoriasis. *J Immunol.* 2010;185:5688-5691.

39 Lowes MA, Kikuchi T, Fuentes-Duculan J, et al. Psoriasis vulgaris lesions contain discrete populations of Th1 and Th17 T cells. *J Invest Dermatol.* 2008;128:1207-1211.

40 Kagami S, Rizzo HL, Lee JJ, Koguchi Y, Blauvelt A. Circulating Th17, Th22, and Th1 cells are increased in psoriasis. *J Invest Dermatol.* 2010;130:1373-1383.

41 McGeachy MJ, Chen Y, Tato CM, et al. The interleukin 23 receptor is essential for the terminal differentiation of interleukin 17-producing effector T helper cells in vivo. *Nat Immunol.* 2009;10:314-324.

42 Lang KS, Recher M, Junt T, et al. Toll-like receptor engagement converts T-cell autoreactivity into overt autoimmune disease. *Nat Med.* 2005;11:138-145.

43 Tonel G, Conrad C. Interplay between keratinocytes and immune cells–recent insights into psoriasis pathogenesis. *Int J Biochem Cell Biol.* 2009;41:963-968.

44 Zheng Y, Danilenko DM, Valdez P, et al. Interleukin-22, a T(H)17 cytokine, mediates IL-23-induced dermal inflammation and acanthosis. *Nature.* 2007;445:648-651.

45 Tohyama M, Yang L, Hanakawa Y, Dai X, Shirakata Y, Sayama K. IFN-alpha enhances IL-22 receptor expression in keratinocytes: a possible role in the development of psoriasis. *J Invest Dermatol.* 2012;132:1933-1935.

46 Eyerich S, Eyerich K, Pennino D, et al. Th22 cells represent a distinct human T cell subset involved in epidermal immunity and remodeling. *J Invest Dermatol.* 2009;119:3573-3585.

47 Liang SC, Tan XY, Luxenberg DP, Karim R, Dunussi-Joannopoulos K, Collins M, et al. Interleukin (IL)-22 and IL-17 are coexpressed by Th17 cells and cooperatively enhance expression of antimicrobial peptides. *J Exp Med*. 2006;203:2271-2279.

48 Wolk K, Kunz S, Witte E, Friedrich M, Asadullah K, Sabat R. IL-22 increases the innate immunity of tissues. *Immunity*. 2004;21:241-254.

49 Peric M, Koglin S, Kim SM, et al. IL-17A enhances vitamin D3-induced expression of cathelicidin antimicrobial peptide in human keratinocytes. *J Immunol*. 2008;181:8504-8512.

50 Conrad C, Meller S, Gilliet M. Plasmacytoid dendritic cells in the skin: to sense or not to sense nucleic acids. *Semin Immunol*. 2009;21:101-109.

51 Sutton CE, Lalor SJ, Sweeney CM, Brereton CF, Lavelle EC, Mills KH. Interleukin-1 and IL-23 induce innate IL-17 production from gammadelta T cells, amplifying Th17 responses and autoimmunity. *Immunity*. 2009;31:331-341.

52 Cai Y, Shen X, Ding C, et al. Pivotal role of dermal IL-17-producing gammadelta T cells in skin inflammation. *Immunity*. 2011;35:596-610.

53 Sumaria N, Roediger B, Ng LG, et al. Cutaneous immunosurveillance by self-renewing dermal gammadelta T cells. *J Exp Med*. 2011;208:505-518.

54 Laggner U, Di Meglio P, Perera GK, et al. Identification of a novel proinflammatory human skin-homing Vγ9Vδ2 T cell subset with a potential role in psoriasis. *J Immunol*. 2011;187:2783-2793.

55 Gladman DD, Farewell VT, Pellett F, Schentag C, Rahman P. HLA is a candidate region for psoriatic arthritis. evidence for excessive HLA sharing in sibling pairs. *Hum Immunol*. 2003;64:887-889.

56 Bhalerao J, Bowcock AM. The genetics of psoriasis: a complex disorder of the skin and immune system. *Hum Mol Genet*. 1998;7:1537-1545.

57 Bluett J, Barton A. What have genome-wide studies told us about psoriatic arthritis? *Curr Rheumatol Rep*. 2012;14:364-368.

58 Jadon D, Tillett W, Wallis D, et al. Exploring ankylosing spondylitis-associated ERAP1, IL23R and IL12B gene polymorphisms in subphenotypes of psoriatic arthritis. *Rheumatology (Oxford)*. 2013;52:261-266.

59 Davidovici BB, Sattar N, Jorg PC, Puig L, Emery P, Barker JN, van de Kerkhof P, Stahle M, Nestle FO, Girolomoni G, Krueger JG for PEARLS. Psoriasis and systemic inflammatory diseases: potential mechanistic links between skin disease and co-morbid conditions. J Invest Dermatol. 2010;130:1785-96.

60 Punzi L, Pianon M, Rizzi E, Rossini P, Todesco S. [Prevalence of post-traumatic psoriatic rheumatism]. *Presse Med*. 1997;26:420.

61 Scarpa R, Del Puente A, di Girolamo C, della Valle G, Lubrano E, Oriente P. Interplay between environmental factors, articular involvement, and HLA-B27 in patients with psoriatic arthritis. *Ann Rheum Dis*. 1992;51:78-79.

62 Pattison E, Harrison BJ, Griffiths CE, Silman AJ, Bruce IN. Environmental risk factors for the development of psoriatic arthritis: results from a case-control study. *Ann Rheum Dis*. 2008;67:672-676.

63 Njobvu P, McGill P. Psoriatic arthritis and human immunodeficiency virus infection in Zambia. *J Rheumatol*. 2000;27:1699-1702.

64 Taglione E, Vatteroni ML, Martini P, et al. Hepatitis C virus infection: prevalence in psoriasis and psoriatic arthritis. *J Rheumatol*. 1999;26:370-372.

65 Gao W, Sweeney C, Walsh C, et al. Notch signalling pathways mediate synovial angiogenesis in response to vascular endothelial growth factor and angiopoietin 2. *Ann Rheum Dis*. 2013;72:1080-1088.

66 Szodoray P, Alex P, Chappell-Woodward CM, et al. Circulating cytokines in Norwegian patients with psoriatic arthritis determined by a multiplex cytokine array system. *Rheumatology (Oxford)*. 2007;46:417-425.

67 Bond SJ, Farewell VT, Schentag CT, et al. Predictors for radiological damage in psoriatic arthritis: results from a single centre. *Ann Rheum Dis*. 2007;66:370-376.

68 Anandarajah AP, Schwarz EM, Totterman S, et al. The effect of etanercept on osteoclast precursor frequency and enhancing bone marrow oedema in patients with psoriatic arthritis. *Ann Rheum Dis*. 2008;67:296-301.

69 Jevtic V, Watt I, Rozman B, Kos-Golja M, Demsar F, Jarh O. Distinctive radiological features of small hand joints in rheumatoid arthritis and seronegative spondyloarthritis demonstrated by contrast-enhanced (Gd-DTPA) magnetic resonance imaging. *Skeletal Radiol*. 1995;24:351-355.

70 McGonagle D, Conaghan PG, Emery P. Psoriatic arthritis: a unified concept twenty years on.[see comment][erratum appears in Arthritis Rheum. 1999;42:1997]. *Arthritis Rheum*. 1999;42:1080-1086.

71 Blau RH, Kaufman RL. Erosive and subluxing cervical spine disease in patients with psoriatic arthritis. *J Rheumatol*. 1987;14:111-117.

72 Salvarani C, Macchioni P, Cremonesi T, et al. The cervical spine in patients with psoriatic arthritis: a clinical, radiological and immunogenetic study. *Ann Rheum Dis*. 1992;51:73-77.

73 Kaplan D, Plotz CM, Nathanson L, Frank L. Cervical Spine in psoriasis and in psoriatic arthritis. *Ann Rheum Dis*. 1964;23:50-56.

Chapter 3

Clinical presentation of psoriasis and psoriatic arthritis

Rebecca I Hartman and Alexa B Kimball

Psoriasis

Plaque psoriasis: clinical presentation, and course

The classic and most common presentation of psoriasis is plaque psoriasis, found in approximately 80–90% of patients. The psoriatic plaque is well-demarcated, erythematous, and scaly (Figure 3.1). The scale is dry, silvery, and has been described as micaceous because it is layered and peels in sheets. Centrally, the scale is adherent and when removed, produces pinpoint bleeding due to dilated superficial capillaries, termed the 'Auspitz sign'. The lesions are often pruritic, but the intensity of the pruritus may vary substantially from patient to patient. Over time, smaller plaques may grow and coalesce into larger lesions. Treatment may cause initial central clearing, resulting in annular plaques. Upon resolution, post-inflammatory hypo- or hyperpigmentation can occur, but scarring is uncommon. Plaque psoriasis is often symmetrical in distribution and favors extensor surfaces, such as the elbows and knees, although it can occur anywhere on the body, including the genitals. The scalp and intergluteal cleft are other common sites of involvement. In addition, the disease may be limited to the palms and soles as in palmoplantar psoriasis.

Plaque psoriasis is typically a chronic disease, and spontaneous remission is rare. The disease may wax and wane, and seasonal variation is

© Springer International Publishing Switzerland 2016
R. Warren and A. Menter (eds.), *Handbook of Psoriasis
and Psoriatic Arthritis*, DOI 10.1007/978-3-319-18227-8_3

17

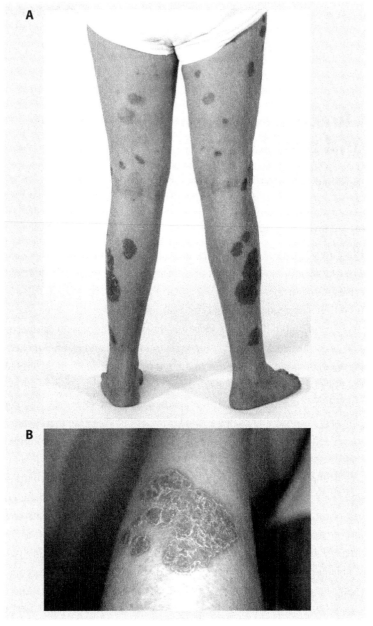

Figure 3.1 Plaque psoriasis. (A) Plaque psoriasis on the lower body. (B) Psoriatic plaques with well-demarcated erythema and adherent silvery scale.

common with improvement in the summer and worsening in the winter. Plaques can remain in specific anatomical sites for years, and the disease tends to recur in these same sites after treatment discontinuation [1]. One-third of patients experience the Koebner phenomenon in which cutaneous trauma to non-lesional skin induces the development of new psoriatic lesions [2].

Other clinical phenotypes

Four additional variants beyond classic plaque psoriasis exist, and include the following: guttate, inverse, pustular, and erythrodermic.

Guttate psoriasis

Guttate psoriasis is a distinct variant of psoriasis consisting of small (less than 1 cm) drop-like pink scaly papules that present in an eruptive fashion on the trunk and proximal extremities (Figure 3.2). Although rare in general, this phenotype is more common in children and young adults. It is often preceded by a bacterial infection, particularly group A streptococcal pharyngitis and sometimes responds to treatment with antibiotics that presumably reduce the triggering antigen [3].

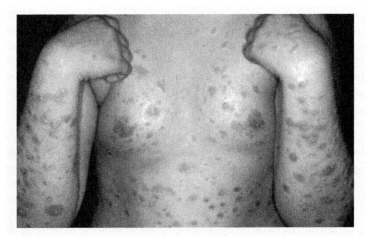

Figure 3.2 Guttate psoriasis. Guttate psoriasis in a child with eruptive drop-like small erythematous scaly papules, a presentation of psoriasis associated with group A streptococcal pharyngitis.

Approximately one in three patients with guttate psoriasis will go on to develop chronic plaque psoriasis [4].

Inverse psoriasis

Inverse psoriasis is localized to the skin folds and presents with well-demarcated, thin erythematous plaques in flexural sites, such as the axillae, groin, neck, and inframammary folds. As these areas are moist, inverse psoriasis lacks the classic dry scale of plaque psoriasis and as a result, may appear shiny.

Pustular psoriasis

Pustular psoriasis is characterized by sterile pustules on an erythematous base. The Von Zumbusch pattern is a rare and life-threatening subtype in which pustules erupt abruptly throughout the body, coalescing into lakes of pus. The eruption may be triggered by withdrawal of systemic corticosteroids. Systemic symptoms often occur, including fever, dehydration, hepatitis, and pneumonitis [5]. Eruptive generalized pustular psoriasis rarely occurs in pregnancy, known as impetigo herpetiformis. Less severe, localized pustular psoriasis subtypes also exist, including a variant limited to the palms and soles (palmoplantar pustular psoriasis) and one limited to the distal digits (acrodermatitis continua of Hallopeau).

Erythrodermic psoriasis

Erythrodermic psoriasis is a rare and severe variant that consists of generalized erythema of at least 90% of the total body surface area (Figure 3.3). Patients typically have a history of chronic psoriasis that is poorly controlled. Systemic steroid use can be a precipitating factor as can severe emotional stress and preceding illness [6]. Erythrodermic psoriasis often requires hospitalization and initiation of systemic therapy given the risk of systemic complications, including fever, infection, dehydration, and high-output heart failure [7].

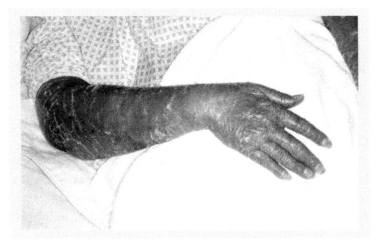

Figure 3.3 Erythrodermic psoriasis. Arm of a hospitalized patient with erythroderma (> 90% BSA involvement) due to poorly controlled psoriasis. BSA, body surface area.

Psoriatic arthritis

Clinical presentation and course

An inflammatory seronegative arthritis occurs in approximately one in three patients with psoriasis, developing 10 years on average after the appearance of skin lesions [8]. The typical primary presentation is an asymmetric mono- or oligoarticular arthritis. The affected joints are painful and may appear red, warm, and swollen. Common sites of involvement include the hands, feet, and spine. Distal joint involvement is frequent and often occurs in a 'ray' pattern, affecting all of the joints in a single digit rather than the same individual joints bilaterally, as seen in rheumatoid arthritis (RA) [8]. Patients may report associated fatigue, morning stiffness, and decreased mobility and function, in particular when using their hands and walking. The arthritis can be erosive, causing clinical joint deformities in 40% of patients [9] and radiographic damage in half of patients [10]. The majority of patients will experience involvement of additional joints over time with the highest rate of progression in the first year of disease [11]. Risk factors for progression include a greater number of inflamed joints, elevated erythrocyte sedimentation rate (ESR), joint damage (clinically or radiographically), and loss of function [12]. Timely diagnosis and treatment can slow joint disease progression [13].

There is an association between more severe skin involvement and the development of arthritis, but no link between the severity of the two disease processes has been found [14]. Arthritis is more common in patients with scalp and intergluteal cleft skin disease as well as those with psoriatic nail disease [15]. Rarely, joint disease can occur in the absence of skin involvement.

Clinical subtypes

There are five subtypes of psoriatic arthritis (PsA) categorized by the location of joint involvement: asymmetrical oligoarticular arthritis, symmetrical polyarthritis, distal interphalangeal arthropathy, arthritis mutilans, and spondylitis with or without sacroiliitis (Table 3.1) [16]. Of note, subtypes may overlap clinically, and they can also change over time, particularly oligoarthritis to polyarthritis [11]. As a result, data on the relative prevalence of each subset vary, but the two most common patterns are peripheral oligo- and polyarthritis [17].

Asymmetrical oligoarticular arthritis

In asymmetrical oligoarticular arthritis, fewer than five small or large joints are affected, most frequently small joints in the hands and feet

Subtype	Approximate frequency at presentation (%)	Clinical features
Asymmetrical oligoarticular	50*	<5 small or large joints, often in the hands, knees, and feet
Symmetrical polyarthritis	35*	≥5 small, medium, or large joints, mimics RA but negative serologies
Distal interphalangeal arthropathy†	<5	Distal interphalangeal joint(s), coexistent nail psoriasis
Arthritis mutilans	<5	Deformities in hands and feet, digital telescoping
Spondylitis +/- sacroiliitis†	<5	Spinal stiffness and pain +/- alternating buttock pain, can be clinically silent

Table 3.1 Psoriatic arthritis subtypes. *Later in disease, asymmetrical oligoarticular and symmetrical polyarthritis have frequencies of approximately 25% and 60%, respectively. †Features of these subtypes may also exist in the asymmetrical oligoarticular and symmetrical polyarthritis subtypes. Adapted with permission from © John Wiley & Sons, 2010. All rights reserved. Cantini et al [17]. Adapted with permission from © Springer Science+Business Media, LLC, 2013. All rights reserved. Dhir and Aggarwal [18].

as well as large joints in the lower limbs. Asymmetrical knee disease is common, and PsA is reportedly the most frequent cause of isolated unilateral knee arthritis in patients under 50 years of age [17]. Symmetry in PsA is a function of the number of inflamed joints, and thus, asymmetric oligoarticular arthritis can progress to symmetric polyarthritis [19]. The symmetric polyarticular subtype affects five or more small, medium, or large joints and can mimic RA clinically, but serologic studies are typically negative.

Distal interphalangeal arthropathy
Distal interphalangeal (DIP) arthropathy predominantly affects the DIP joints and often coexists with psoriatic nail disease. DIP involvement is a distinguishing feature of PsA that differentiates it from other erosive arthritides, such as rheumatoid arthritis. Although DIP joint involvement is present in nearly half of patients with psoriatic arthritis, the DIP predominant subtype occurs relatively infrequently [9].

Arthritis mutilans
Arthritis mutilans is a rare variant characterized by rapidly progressive severe joint deformities of the hands and feet due to osteolysis (Figure 3.4). Clinical findings include shortened digits with excess skin folds, joint hypermobility, and digital telescoping. The latter is also known as opera glass finger or 'doigt en lorgnette'.

Spondylitis
Although spondylitis or vertebral inflammation occurs in 40% of patients with psoriatic arthritis, only 5% of patients have predominantly axial involvement [16]. Axial disease is more common in males and may occur with or without sacroiliitis (involvement of the sacroiliac joint). Spondylitis presents clinically with spinal stiffness and pain, while sacroiliitis causes alternating buttock pain [17]. However, one in four patients with axial disease have no clinical symptoms [20]. Compared with other spondyloarthropathies, such as ankylosing spondylitis (AS), PsA more commonly exhibits asymmetrical sacroiliitis and cervical spine disease; the lumbar spine is involved less frequently [21]. Syndesmophyte

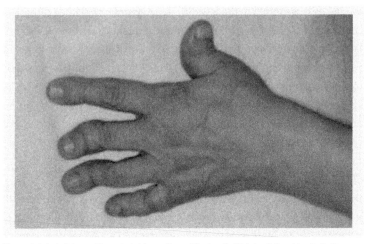

Figure 3.4 Arthritis mutilans. Arthritis mutilans of the hand with joint deformities, including digital shortening and telescoping of the third digit. Published with kind permission of © M. Alora-Palli, 2014. All rights reserved).

formation, bony growth within the spinal ligaments, can also occur in psoriatic spondylitis and cause vertebral fusion [20]. Symptoms often improve over time, most likely due to treatment [20]. However, radiographic progression is common; one study found that half of arthritic patients developed a new diagnosis of radiographic sacroiliitis over a 10 year period [20]. Nevertheless, psoriatic spondylitis typically has a milder course and better prognosis than AS [17].

Associated clinical findings

Nail disease occurs in approximately half of all psoriatic patients, and is the only cutaneous manifestation in a small fraction of patients. Nail involvement is more common in patients with psoriatic arthritis, likely due to the close anatomic proximity of the nail unit and distal phalanx [14]. Psoriasis can involve the nail matrix as well as the nail bed. Signs of nail matrix involvement include pitting and leukonychia (white spots on the nail plate). Nail bed disease can cause subungual hyperkeratosis, onycholysis (distal separation of the nail plate from the nail bed), and oil drops (round yellow discolorations of the nail bed).

In comparison to skin disease, nail psoriasis responds to therapy more slowly and is more recalcitrant to topical therapy.

PsA can also cause soft tissue inflammation. Enthesitis, inflammation at the insertion sites of ligaments and tendons to bones, may occur and cause edema and pain. The pelvis, Achilles tendon, and plantar fascia are most commonly affected. Patients can also develop tendon sheath inflammation or tenosynovitis, often in the finger flexor and Achilles tendons. A combination of digital arthritis, enthesitis, and tenosynovitis causes dactylitis, also known as 'sausage digit', in which there is diffuse swelling of a digit, more frequently a toe than a finger [22]. Dactylitis is a cardinal feature of PsA that is present in nearly half of patients, but rarely seen in RA [22]. Additionally, some patients with PsA experience swelling of distal extremities and pitting edema, either as a feature of previously diagnosed disease, or less commonly, as the initial manifestation [23].

Approximately one in three patients with PsA will have ocular inflammation on exam, a finding that is more common in patients with joint disease [24]. Ocular involvement often occurs after the development of arthritis and can cause conjunctivitis, episcleritis, and uveitis [25]. Acute uveitis typically presents with eye redness, pain, photophobia, and blurry vision, but psoriatic uveitis can occur insidiously with worsening vision as the only initial symptom [25]. As a result, eye complaints warrant prompt ophthalmologic evaluation, and regular eye exams are recommended for patients with psoriasis [25].

References

1 Clark RA. Gone but not forgotten: lesional memory in psoriatic skin. *J Invest Dermatol.* 2011;131:283-285.
2 Melsky JW, Bernhard JD, Stern RS. The Koebner (isomorphic) response in psoriasis: associations with early age at onset and multiple previous therapies. *Arch Dermatol.* 1983;119:655-659.
3 Telfer NR, Chalmers RJ, Whale K, Coleman G. The role of streptococcal infection in the initiation of guttate psoriasis. *Arch Dermatol.* 1992;128:39-42.
4 Martin BA, Chalmers RJ, Telfer NR. How great is the risk of further psoriasis following a single episode of acute guttate psoriasis? *Arch Dermatol.* 199;132:717-718.
5 Varman KM, Namias N, Schulman CI, Pizano LR. Acute generalized pustular psoriasis, von Zumbusch type, treated in the burn unit. A review of clinical features and new therapeutics. *Burns.* 2014;40:35-39.
6 Boyd AS, Menter A. Erythrodermic psoriasis: precipitating factors, course, and prognosis in 50 patients. *JAMA.* 1989;21:985-991.
7 Rosenbach M, Hsu S, Korman NJ, et al. Treatment of erythrodermic psoriasis: from the medical board of the National Psoriasis Foundation. *J Am Acad Dermatol.* 2010;62:655-662.

8 Gladman DD, Antoni C, Mease P, Clegg DO, Nash P. Psoriatic arthritis: epidemiology, clinical features, course, and outcome. *Ann Rheum Dis*. 2005;64:ii14–ii17.

9 Veale D, Rogers S, Fitzgerald O. Classification of clinical subsets in psoriatic arthritis. *Br J Rheumatol*. 1994;33(2):133-138.

10 Kane D, Stafford L, Bresnihan B, Fitzgerald O. A prospective, clinical and radiological study of early psoriatic arthritis: an early synovitis clinic experience. *Rheumatology (Oxford)*. 2003;42:1460-1468.

11 McHugh NJ, Balachrishnan C, Jones SM. Progression of peripheral joint disease in psoriatic arthritis: a 5-yr prospective study. *Rheumatology (Oxford)*. 2003;42:778-783.

12 Ritchlin CT, Kavanaugh A, Gladman DD, et al. Treatment recommendations for psoriatic arthritis. *Ann Rheum Dis*. 2009;68:1387-1394.

13 Gladman DD, Thavaneswaran A, Chandran V, Cook RJ. Do patients with psoriatic arthritis who present early fare better than those presenting later in the disease? *Ann Rheum Dis*. 2011;70:2152-2154.

14 Reich K, Krüger K, Mössner R, Augustin M. Epidemiology and clinical pattern of psoriatic arthritis in Germany: a prospective interdisciplinary epidemiological study of 1511 patients with plaque-type psoriasis. *Br J Dermatol*. 2009;160:1040-1047.

15 Wilson FC, Icen M, Crowson CS, McEvoy MT, Gabriel SE, Kremers HM. Incidence and clinical predictors of psoriatic arthritis in patients with psoriasis: a population-based study. *Arthritis Rheum*. 2009;61:233-239.

16 Moll JM, Wright V. Psoriatic arthritis. *Semin Arthritis Rheum*. 1973;3:55-78.

17 Cantini F, Niccoli L, Nannini C, Kaloudi O, Bertoni M, Cassarà E. Psoriatic arthritis: a systematic review. *Int J Rheum Dis*. 2010;13:300-317.

18 Dhir V, Aggarwal A. Psoriatic arthritis: a critical review. *Clin Rev Allergy Immunol*. 2013;44: 141-148.

19 Helliwell PS, Hetthen J, Sokoll K, et al. Joint symmetry in early and late rheumatoid and psoriatic arthritis: comparison with a mathematical model. *Arthritis Rheum*. 2000;43:865-871.

20 Chandran V, Barrett J, Schentag CT, Farewell VT, Gladman DD. Axial psoriatic arthritis: update on a longterm prospective study. *J Rheumatol*. 2009;36:2744-2750.

21 Helliwell PS, Taylor WJ. Classification and diagnostic criteria for psoriatic arthritis. *Ann Rheum Dis*. 2005;64:ii3-ii8.

22 Brockbank JE, Stein M, Schentag CT, Gladman DD. Dactylitis in psoriatic arthritis: a marker for disease severity? *Ann Rheum Dis*. 2005;64:188-190.

23 Cantini F, Salvarani C, Olivieri I, et al. Distal extremity swelling with pitting edema in psoriatic arthritis: a case-control study. *Clin Exp Rheumatol*. 2001;19:291-296.

24 Lambert JR, Wright V. Eye inflammation in psoriatic arthritis. *Ann Rheum Dis*. 1976;35:354-356.

25 Au SC, Yaniv S, Gottlieb AB. Psoriatic eye manifestations. *Psoriasis Forum*. 2011;17:169-179.

Chapter 4

Diagnosis and evaluation of psoriasis and psoriatic arthritis

Eric Ruderman and Kenneth B Gordon

The most critical element in the diagnosis of psoriasis and psoriatic arthritis (PsA) is understanding that it is a clinical diagnosis. In a patient with joint pain and/or swelling the differentiation of PsA from other types of inflammatory arthritis may be a central element in treatment decisions. Unfortunately, there are often no specific laboratory or radiographic findings that reliably confirm this challenging diagnosis. Thus, it is the cumulative evidence derived from the patient evaluation, including a combination of history, clinical exam, laboratory findings, and imaging that lead to an appropriate diagnosis of psoriasis and/or PsA.

History

The medical history taken from the patient can often identify a likely case of PsA even before the physical exam. As one of the principle indicators of psoriatic arthritis is the presence or history of cutaneous psoriasis, establishing the skin diagnosis is one of the initial tasks in taking a clinical history. Most patients will present with skin disease long before they develop joint disease, and this pre-existing psoriasis can suggest a diagnosis of psoriatic arthritis. However, one must always remember that up to 10% of patients will present with joint symptoms before developing skin psoriasis. Moreover, in a small subset of patients, there may never have been

© Springer International Publishing Switzerland 2016
R. Warren and A. Menter (eds.), *Handbook of Psoriasis and Psoriatic Arthritis*, DOI 10.1007/978-3-319-18227-8_4

a specific diagnosis of psoriasis, so careful questioning for any history of scaly rash or nail changes is important. A history of severe dandruff, for example, may be indicative of scalp psoriasis that has never been formally diagnosed. If a personal history of psoriasis is not evident, a full family history may be critical. The Classification Criteria for Psoriatic Arthritis (CASPAR, see below) identifies a family history of psoriasis as an important element in the diagnosis of PsA. Finally, a personal or family history of other potentially related conditions may be important. Of particular note are spondyloarthropathy features in other organ systems, including uveitis or colitis, which may be helpful in identifying a potential diagnosis of PsA in a patient with inflammatory joint symptoms.

The patient's history of musculoskeletal symptoms may provide helpful clues in diagnosing PsA. Application of the CASPAR criteria begins by establishing a history of inflammatory joint disease, but this history may include peripheral, axial, or entheseal involvement [1]. Enthesitis refers to inflammation at the insertion of the tendon or ligament into bone. This is not always within the joint space as enthesitis can occur at a considerable distance from the joints, in sites such as on the pelvic brim or at the greater trochanter. As with other spondyloarthropathies, enthesitis is a common feature of PsA; patients may present with enthesitis alone, such as plantar fasciitis or Achilles tendonitis, or with no other evidence of arthritis. Even areas that are infrequently considered in the evaluation of inflammatory arthritis may be important. For example, PsA may occasionally present with chest wall pain, with the pain presumably arising from entheseal insertions in the spine, sternum, or ribs. The synovitis of PsA is clinically similar to other types of inflammatory arthritis, but PsA patients may have fewer joints involved than in rheumatoid arthritis (RA), and they may present with asymmetrical or predominantly lower extremity involvement. As in all types of inflammatory arthritis, morning stiffness, either peripheral or axial, is an important component of PsA and should be queried and quantified. Morning stiffness lasting more than 30–60 minutes is a particularly important finding in the diagnosis of PsA.

Joint exam

The second element of the evaluation of PsA is an objective assessment of joint and entheseal involvement. Formal joint counts may be assessed by examining either 28 joints (upper extremities and knees only) or a greater number of joints for swelling and tenderness; these are the same joint counts that are used in the evaluation of RA. The more extensive joint count may be particularly useful in PsA, as it may identify lower extremity or distal interphalangeal (DIP) involvement that might otherwise be missed. Such joint counts are used commonly in clinical trials but are also useful in clinical practice to provide an objective measurement of joint involvement. Joint counts also form an important component of the composite outcome measurements discussed below. While formal joint counts are particularly useful for following the course of a patient with PsA, simply identifying the presence and general extent of synovitis may be enough to make the diagnosis. The two key findings in a joint with synovitis are swelling and tenderness. Tenderness may be elicited by querying the patient while applying firm pressure on the joint; in deeper joints, such as the shoulder or hip, pain experienced during passive range of motion may also indicate synovitis. Swelling may be subtle, and can sometimes be identified as bogginess or soft tissue swelling that is more prominent than the contralateral joint.

The 28 joint count, which includes metacarpophalangeal and proximal interphalangeal joints, wrists, elbows, shoulders, and knees is the most practical joint count used in clinical practice (Figure 4.1A). It may be easily performed with the patient sitting in the exam room rather than lying down on an exam table, and it does not require that they remove their shoes (although examination of the feet is still important for patients who report lower extremity symptoms). It should be remembered that the standard 28 joint count used in disease activity scores does not include the DIP joints, which may be involved in PsA and should be assessed separately. More extensive joint counts, which include the DIP joints, are more commonly used in clinical trials than in clinical practice (Figure 4.1B). In addition to the DIP joints, more extensive joint counts include the temperomandibular, acromioclavicular, sternoclavicular, hip,

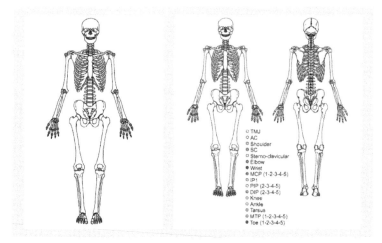

Figure 4.1 Joints assessed in a standard 28 joint count (A) and 66 joint count (B). Reproduced with permission from © Professional Communications Inc, 2013. All rights reserved. Terkeltaub R, Edwards NL. Gout: Diagnosis and Management of Gouty Arthritis and Hyperuricemia, 3rd ed. West Islip, NY: Professional Communications, Inc; 2013. Terkeltaub and Edwards [2].

ankle, tarsal, metatarsophalangeal, and the interphalangeal joints of the feet, although the hips are assessed only for tenderness and not swelling.

Entheseal exam

A careful examination for the presence of entheseal tenderness should be part of the evaluation of a patient with PsA. As previously noted, common locations for entheseal tenderness include the Achilles tendon insertions, the plantar fascia, the medial and lateral epicondyles, the inferior patella, and tendon insertions at the trochanters. If tenderness is evoked with palpation of these areas, it may indicate a diagnosis of PsA.

While a general examination of these entheseal sites may suffice in clinical practice, there have been efforts to quantify this evaluation for use in clinical trials [3]. There are several standardized measures that have been used in clinical trials and epidemiological studies. These range from the Mander Enthesitis Index (MEI), which was originally developed for assessing enthesitis in ankylosing spondylitis (AS) and assesses 66 unique entheseal insertion sites, to the more simplified Leeds Enthesitis Index (LEI), which focuses on bilateral evaluation at just six sites (lateral epicondyles, medial femoral condyles, and Achilles insertion), and was developed specifically for use in PsA. While formal enthesitis assessments are not routinely carried out in clinical practice, it is important to note changes in the extent of this feature with changes in therapy.

Examination for dactylitis

Examination for the presence and extent of dactylitis, or 'sausage digits', should be part of the initial evaluation of PsA, and these findings can be followed during the course of the disease. Dactylitis is presumed to result from swelling of both the joints and the tendons in the involved finger or toe. The finding of tenderness in a dactylitic digit may be more indicative of active disease than the chronic, non-tender swelling that can sometimes occur. While efforts have been made to define quantifiable indices for dactylitis [3], it may be sufficient, both in clinical trials and clinical practice, to simply note the number of involved digits.

Axial evaluation

Axial involvement of PsA can be one of the most significant but challenging parts of the evaluation. Unfortunately, there are no specific tools for evaluating axial disease in PsA. Diagnosis of axial disease is generally made on the basis of the patient's medical history, with pain and morning stiffness being the primary associated findings. Tenderness can be elicited but other physical signs are extremely difficult to assess. As with enthesitis, outcomes developed for use in AS, although not specifically validated for this disease, have been applied to axial PsA. In particular, mobility measurements used in AS may be helpful for monitoring axial disease in PsA.

The Schober's test is used to measure mobility at the lumbar spine (Figure 4.2). The Schober test is performed by marking one line between the posterior superior iliac spines and a second line 10 cm above this on an individual standing erect The patient is then asked to bend forward and the distance between the two lines is measured again; with normal lumbar flexion, the distance between the two marks should extend to approximately 15 cm as the skin stretches over the spine. In patients with

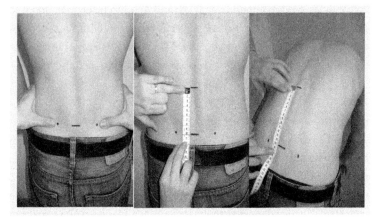

Figure 4.2 The Schober test to assess mobility at the lumbar spine. Reproduced with permission from © BMJ Publishing Group, 2009. All rights reserved. Sieper et al [4].

limited mobility, from AS, axial PsA, or other axial spondyloarthropathies, the distance will be less than 14 cm.

A second measure of axial mobility is the occiput to wall test, where the distance between the posterior occiput and the wall is measured in a patient standing with their heels up against a wall. Patients with normal cervical extension should be able to touch their occiput to the wall easily; the distance is increased as cervical mobility diminishes. Occiput to wall distance is generally increased only in late-stage AS.

In clinical practice, simple measures of axial function, such as the ability to turn one's head and look to the rear when backing up a car, are useful parameters to assess and follow.

Nail changes

Nail changes are common in psoriasis, but are particularly common in PsA, with up to 80% of patients with PsA having some of the nail changes that are described elsewhere in this text. Evaluation of a patient with PsA should include documentation of specific nails involved, in both hands and feet. There is a quantifiable assessment of nail involvement, the Nail Psoriasis Severity Index (NAPSI) that may be useful when a quantifiable measurement is desired, such as in clinical trials or registries (Table 4.1) [5].

Laboratory testing

There are no laboratory tests that are useful in making a specific diagnosis of PsA. Laboratory tests may give hints to help distinguish PsA from other forms of inflammatory arthritis, such as RA, or in evaluating the activity of disease, but they are rarely of any real diagnostic value. Rheumatoid factor (RF) is usually negative in PsA (indeed, a negative RF is one element of the CASPAR criteria) but a positive RF may be seen in as many as 10% of patients [6]. A false positive RF is more common in older individuals in general, so a positive RF test does not necessarily exclude PsA in this group. The presence of antibodies to cyclic citrullinated peptides (anti-CCP or ACPA) may help distinguish polyarticular RA from PsA, as they are generally considered to be more specific for RA than a positive RF. However, anti-CCP antibodies have been reported in patients with PsA, so their presence does not completely rule out the diagnosis [7,8].

Elevated acute-phase reactants, either sedimentation rate or C-reactive protein (CRP), non-specific indicators of inflammation, may be seen in one-third of patients with PsA, but less frequently than in RA [6]. As a

---

The Nail Psoriasis Severity Index

The nail is divided with imaginary horizontal and longitudinal lines into quadrants. Each nail is given a score for nail bed psoriasis (0–4) and nail matrix psoriasis (0–4) depending on the presence of any of the features of nail psoriasis in that quadrant.

1. Evaluation 1: Nail matrix

In each quadrant of the nail, nail matrix psoriasis is evaluated by presence of any of the nail matrix features (pitting, leukonychia red spots in the lunula, and/or crumbling): 0 for none, 1 if present in 1 quadrant of the nail, 2 if present in 2 quadrants of the nail, 3 if present in 3 quadrants of the nail, and 4 if present in 4 quadrants of the nail.

2. Evaluation 2: Nail bed

Nail bed psoriasis is evaluated by the presence of any of the nail bed features (onycholysis, splinter hemorrhages, subungual hyperkeratosis, and/or 'oil drop' [salmon patch dyschroma]): 0 for none, 1 for 1 quadrant only, 2 for 2 quadrants, 3 for 3 quadrants, and 4 for 4 quadrants.

3. Each nail gets a matrix score and a nail bed score, the total of which is the score for that nail (0–8).

4. Each nail is evaluated, and the sum of all the nails is the total NAPSI score. The sum of the scores from all nails is 0–80 or 0–160 if toenails are included. At any time the matrix or nail bed score can be assessed independently if desired.

If a target nail scale is desired, the same technique can be used to evaluate all 8 parameters (pitting, leukonychia, red spots in lunula, crumbling, oil drop, onycholysis, hyperkeratosis, and/or splinter hemorrhages) in each quadrant of the nail, giving that 1 nail a score of 0–32.

Table 4.1 Grading psoriatic nails using the National Psoriasis Severity Index. NAPSI, Nail Psoriasis Severity Index. Adapted from © American Academy of Dermatology, 2003. All rights reserved. Rich et al [6].

consequence, these tests are generally not as helpful as biomarkers of disease activity in PsA as they are in RA.

Human leukocyte antigen (HLA)-B27 positivity may be seen in patients with PsA. It is more common in those with axial disease and occurs less frequently in patients with strictly peripheral disease (although it is still more common than in the general population) [9]. Psoriatic skin disease without PsA is not associated with an increased prevalence of HLA-B27 positivity.

Radiographic evaluation

Radiographic changes are not always seen in early PsA but, when present, may be diagnostically useful. In particular, these changes can assist in differentiating PsA from RA or osteoarthritis (OA), as well as indicating the destructive activity of the disease. The radiographic changes seen in RA are those of destructive bony lesions and cartilage loss, with periarticular erosions and joint space narrowing, while radiographs in OA show osteophytes, or evidence of new bone production. PsA has a unique radiographic picture, where both destructive and productive bony changes may be seen in the same joint.

Hand and foot radiographs may be useful as part of the baseline evaluation, along with radiographs of any other involved joints. While erosive disease may be seen, as in RA, radiographic changes in the DIP joints may help to distinguish PsA from RA. In addition, unique radiographic features that may be seen in PsA include periostitis, distal tuft resorption, and soft tissue swelling in digits with dactylitis (Figure 4.3).

Productive changes may be seen as new bone formation develops at entheseal insertions; in severe cases, this may produce a 'pencil-in-cup' deformity, as new bone formation at the base of the distal phalynx surrounds the distal end of the more proximal phalynx, which has eroded away. In clinical trials, a modified version of the Sharp radiographic scoring system that includes DIP joints has been used to monitor radiographic change over time.

In patients with symptoms that suggest spondyloarthritis, axial radiographic changes can also be seen, including the typical syndesmophytes seen in spondyloarthropathies. Pelvic radiographs may show

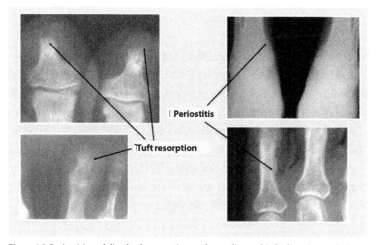

Figure 4.3 Periostitis and distal tuft resorption are key radiographic findings in psoriatic arthritis. Reproduced with permission from © Remedica Medical Education and Publishing, 2014. All rights reserved. Mease and van der Heijde [10].

unilateral sacroiliitis, rather than the bilateral changes typically seen in AS. Radiographic evidence of lumbar spine involvement is less common than in classical AS. The modified Stoke Ankylosing Spondylitis Spinal Score (mSASSS) may be used to follow radiographic change in the cervical and lumbar spine over time.

Other imaging modalities

Beyond plain radiographs, other imaging technologies have been used in PsA. Ultrasound imaging may be used to evaluate enthesitis as well as synovitis within the joints. Computed tomography may be useful in evaluation of joints, such as the sternoclavicular joints or the sacroiliac (SI) joints, as it can be difficult to evaluate properly with plain radiographs. Magnetic resonance imaging (MRI) may be useful in identifying early changes in peripheral joints, but is particularly useful at identifying sacroiliitis; MRI abnormalities in the SI joints may be present years before they can be seen on plain radiographs. Bone marrow edema on MRI, an indication of active inflammation, may be seen even without the use of gadolinium contrast, thus contrast imaging is not generally necessary.

Putting it all together: the diagnosis of psoriatic arthritis

The presence of the clinical symptoms and signs of inflammatory arthritis are, of course, the initial necessary elements to diagnosing PsA. However, even when these elements are present, differentiating PsA from other forms of arthritis may be a challenge. As has been suggested in this chapter, the differential diagnosis of PsA can be quite broad, and includes both inflammatory and non-inflammatory types of arthritis (Table 4.2).

An accurate diagnosis of the type of arthritis is required to ensure that the most appropriate therapy is chosen for the patient, thus making these distinctions is critical for the well-being of patients.

Osteoarthritis

OA is the most common form of arthritis, and must always be a primary consideration, especially in the setting of hand and spine involvement, although OA would be an unusual finding in younger patients. OA in the hands typically involves the DIP joints, and there may be erythema of these joints suggestive of an inflammatory process, but the radiographic findings should be distinguishable from those of PsA. Clinically, nail changes, particularly in those digits with DIP arthritis, may help to identify the diagnosis as PsA rather than OA.

Degenerative arthritis of the spine may cause axial symptoms in patients with concurrent psoriasis. Prolonged morning stiffness, either in peripheral joints or the spine, is not a typical feature of degenerative arthritis and, when present, should prompt consideration of an inflammatory arthritis such as PsA. Radiographic changes in the spine resulting from degenerative disc disease should also be distinguishable

Types of arthritis
Osteoarthritis (DIP involvement)
Rheumatoid arthritis
Axial spondyloarthritis
Reactive arthritis
Gout (monoarthritis or oligoarthritis)

Table 4.2 Types of arthritis to consider when carrying out differential diagnosis of psoriatic arthritis. DIP, distal interphalangeal.

on X-ray from the syndesmophytes and sacroiliitis that can accompany PsA. Radiographically, diffuse idiopathic skeletal hyperostosis (DISH), in which there is calcification of the anterior longitudinal ligaments of the spine, may suggest the syndesmophyte formation that can be seen in PsA, but careful evaluation should be able to distinguish between the two.

Rheumatoid arthritis

Differentiating RA from PsA may prove more challenging, especially in those psoriatic patients with rheumatoid-like polyarticular involvement. Oligoarticular, asymmetrical joint involvement would argue for PsA over RA, as would DIP joint involvement, as these joints are rarely affected in RA. Tendonitis can occur in RA, but prominent symptoms of enthesitis, particularly when joint involvement itself is relatively mild, should prompt consideration of PsA or another spondyloarthropathy. The inflammatory low back pain that can accompany PsA can also help to distinguish it from RA; cervical spine involvement may be seen in RA, but lumbar spine involvement is rare.

Ankylosing spondylitis

Finally, PsA needs to be distinguished from other forms of spondyloarthropathy. A history of inflammatory bowel disease may suggest a diagnosis of irritable bowel disease (IBD)-associated arthropathy, and a recent history of gastrointestinal or genitourinary infection should prompt consideration of reactive arthritis. AS presents with inflammatory low back pain similar to that sometimes seen in PsA, and may also be associated with peripheral arthritis and enthesitis. Radiographic evidence of vertebral ankylosis and bilateral sacroiliitis, as opposed to the unilateral involvement that is more commonly seen in PsA, might suggest this diagnosis of AS [11].

The clinical manifestations of the spondyloarthropathies may overlap considerably. Recognizing this, the Assessment of Spondyloarthritis International Society (ASAS) has developed new classification criteria for axial and peripheral spondyloarthropathies, which are intended to provide a framework for therapy that is based more on symptom complexes than on formal disease definitions [12,13]. The presence of psoriasis is an important component in both sets of criteria. These criteria remain a work in progress, particularly those for peripheral spondyloarthropathy; although some have raised concerns that they threaten to diminish the significance of PsA as a unique discrete entity by blurring the distinction between this diagnosis and the more inclusive diagnosis of spondyloarthropathy.

Classification of psoriatic arthritis: criteria for identification

As is clear from the above discussion, PsA is not always clearly distinct from other forms of arthritis, a fact that has lead to the slow development of clinically useful and accurate classification systems. Historically, PsA was presumed to be simply a variation of RA in patients who also had concurrent psoriasis. Verna Wright first proposed classifying PsA as a distinct clinical entity in the 1950s, and her delineation of the clinical patterns of joint involvement in this disease, first published with John Moll in 1973, remains in widespread use today [3]. With this publication, Moll and Wright divided PsA patients into five distinct patterns of peripheral and axial arthritis (Table 4.3).

Although it is still used, the Moll and Wright scheme for separating PsA patients by pattern of joint involvement has its limitations. Joint involvement may change over time, so that patients may move from one pattern of joint involvement to another. Within this classification scheme, isolated DIP involvement and arthritis mutilans, while both unusual, are the most specific joint findings indicating PsA. In clinical trials, response to therapy does not appear to differ according to patterns of joint involvement, except for axial disease, which is less responsive to non-biologic therapies.

Moll and Wright classifications for psoriatic arthritis
Asymmetric oligoarthritis or monoarthritis of DIP, PIP, or MCP joints
Symmetric polyarthritis resembling RA, with negative rheumatoid factor
Arthritis with DIP joint predominance
Arthritis mutilans
Predominantly axial arthritis, with or without peripheral joint involvement

Table 4.3 Moll and Wright standard early classifications for psoriatic arthritis. DIP, distal interphalangeal; MCP, metacarpophalangeal; PIP, proximal interphalangeal.

Classification of psoriatic arthritis: CASPAR criteria

As specific therapies for PsA are developed, accurate classification of the disease has become increasingly important, as it ensures homogenous patient selection in both trials and in practice. In 2008, The Classification of Psoriatic Arthritis group (CASPAR), a cooperative international effort, reviewed existing classification schemes and developed new criteria for psoriatic arthritis. The CASPAR group applied elements of existing, published criteria to representative cases of PsA, developing a criteria set that is both sensitive and specific for PsA. The CASPAR criteria (Table 4.4), when applied to patients with definite inflammatory joint, axial, or entheseal disease, identify patients with PsA with high specificity [14].

Importantly, the CASPAR criteria are predicated on the presence of inflammatory musculoskeletal disease; without this, the other elements of the criteria set should not be considered, and the disease cannot be classified as PsA. It should also be noted that a current or past diagnosis of psoriasis is a key element of these criteria; current psoriasis is twice as important as any other component. However, a diagnosis of PsA can be made using the CASPAR criteria without a diagnosis of psoriatic skin

Criterion	Description
1. Evidence of psoriasis	
a. Current psoriasis*	Skin or scalp disease, judged by rheumatologist/ dermatologist
b. Personal history of psoriasis	History obtained from patient or health care professional
c. Family history of psoriasis	History in first or second degree relative
2. Psoriatic nail dystrophy	Typical changes on current physical exam, including onycholysis, pitting and hyperkeratosis
3. Negative rheumatoid factor	By any method except latex, according to local reference range
4. Dactylitis	
a. Current	Swelling of an entire digit
b. History	History as recorded by a rheumatologist
5. Radiological evidence of juxtaarticular new bone formation	Ill-defined ossification near the joint margins on plain radiographs of the hands or feet

*Scored as 2 points. A diagnosis of psoriatic arthritis can be made in a patient with inflammatory articular disease (joint, spine, entheseal) who has ≥3 points.

Table 4.4 The classification criteria for psoriatic arthritis. Adapted from © American College of Rheumatology, 2006. All rights reserved. Taylor et al [1].

disease, for example, in a patient with a family history of psoriasis and psoriatic nail disease.

Measurement of psoriatic arthritis for research: composite disease activity scores

In clinical trials, composite measures of disease outcome are commonly used as endpoints to identify response to therapy. The first outcome developed specifically for PsA clinical trials was the Psoriatic Arthritis Response Criteria (PsARC). The PsARC, which uses a combination of patient and physician assessment and counts of tender and swollen joints, was developed as consensus criteria for response in the Veterans Affairs (VA) cooperative sulfasalazine trials during the 1980s. A PsARC response is relatively easy to achieve, however, which can make it difficult to use this measure to identify an active drug in clinical trials, where there is often a high placebo response rate.

In clinical trials for PsA, disease activity scales developed for, and validated in, RA have also been used as outcome measures. The American College of Rheumatology 20 (ACR20) response rate has been used frequently in trials of PsA. Achieving this outcome requires a 20% improvement in both the number of swollen and tender joints, along with a 20% improvement in at least five out of seven other measures of disease activity, including function and levels of acute phase reactants. While useful, the ACR response is an imperfect measurement of response in PsA. Improvement in swollen and tender joints may be difficult to assess in patients with only a few active joints, and the utility of acute phase reactants is limited in a disease in which as many as two out of three patients do not have an elevated sedimentation rate or CRP.

One of the limitations of existing composite measurements is that they do not specifically assess the skin, nail, or entheseal components of PsA. Recently, the Group for the Assessment of Psoriasis and Psoriatic Arthritis (GRAPPA), in conjunction with the Outcomes Measures in Rheumatology (OMERACT) group, has been working to develop a composite measurement of disease activity that is specific to PsA. While still a work in progress, the goal of this instrument will be to assess both the unique manifestations of the joint involvement in PsA and the non-joint manifestations, including dermatologic manifestations, enthesitis, and dactylitis.

Conclusions

An accurate diagnosis of PsA is the first stage towards effective therapy. A thorough history and physical examination is the first step, as much of the diagnosis rests on signs and symptoms. Diagnostic testing and radiographic imaging may be helpful adjuncts, but are never the primary elements of the diagnosis. More recent attempts to classify PsA, particularly with the CASPAR criteria, are helping to differentiate PsA from other forms of inflammatory arthritis and should, ultimately, lead to a better understanding of this unique disease entity. This understanding, in turn, will help produce better clinical outcome measures and, eventually, better and more focused treatments.

References

1 Taylor W, Gladman D, Helliwell P, et al. Classification criteria for psoriatic arthritis: development of new criteria from a large international study. *Arthritis Rheum*. 2006;54:2665-2673.

2 Terkeltaub R, Edwards NL. *Gout: Diagnosis and Management of Gouty Arthritis and Hyperuricemia*, 3rd ed. 2013; West Islip, NY: Professional Communications, Inc.

3 Coates LC, Helliwell PS. Disease measurement--enthesitis, skin, nails, spine and dactylitis. *Best Pract Res Clin Rheumatol*. 2010;24:659-670.

4 Sieper J, Rudwaleit M, Baraliakos X, et al. The Assessment of SpondyloArthritis international Society (ASAS) handbook: a guide to assess spondyloarthritis. *Ann Rheum Dis*. 2009;68:ii1-ii44.

5 Rich P, Scher RK. Nail Psoriasis Severity Index: a useful tool for evaluation of nail psoriasis. *J Am Acad Dermatol*. 2003;49:206-212.

6 Gladman DD. Psoriatic arthritis. *Baillieres Clin Rheumatol*. 1995;9:319-329.

7 Alenius GM, Berglin E, Rantapää Dahlqvist S. Antibodies against cyclic citrullinated peptide (CCP) in psoriatic patients with or without joint inflammation. *Ann Rheum Dis*. 2006;65:398-400.

8 Bogliolo L, Alpini C, Caporali R, Scirè CA, Moratti R, Montecucco C. Antibodies to cyclic citrullinated peptides in psoriatic arthritis. *J Rheumatol*. 2005;32:511-515.

9 Zochling J, Smith EU. Seronegative spondyloarthritis. *Best Pract Res Clin Rheumatol*. 2010;24:747-756.

10 Mease P, van der Heijde D. Joint damage in psoriatic arthritis: how is it assessed and can it be prevented? *Int J Adv Rheumatol*. 2006;4:38-48.

11 Gladman DD. Axial disease in psoriatic arthritis. *Curr Rheumatol Rep*. 2007;9:455-460.

12 Rudwaleit M, Landewé R, van der Heijde D, et al. The development of Assessment of SpondyloArthritis international Society classification criteria for axial spondyloarthritis (part I): classification of paper patients by expert opinion including uncertainty appraisal. *Ann Rheum Dis*. 2009;68:770-776.

13 Rudwaleit M, van der Heijde D, Landewé R.The development of Assessment of SpondyloArthritis international Society classification criteria for axial spondyloarthritis (part II): validation and final selection. *Ann Rheum Dis*. 2009;68:777-83.

14 Garrett S, Jenkinson T, Kennedy LG, Whitelock H, Gaisford P, Calin A. A new approach to defining disease status in ankylosing spondylitis: the Bath Ankylosing Spondylitis Disease Activity Index. *J Rheumatol*. 1994;21:2286-2291.

Chapter 5

Treatment of psoriasis

Matthias Augustin and Marc Alexander Radtke

Strategies for psoriasis management: treatment goals and targeted treatment

Treatment of psoriasis and psoriatic arthritis (PsA) can be challenging since a large variety of clinical conditions, different psoriasis types and patient factors need to be considered. Moreover, in the past decade, a large number of effective treatments have been developed and standards of management were consented. This included evidence-based guidelines (Figure 5.1), implementation tools, and valid outcomes measures.

Another landmark was the international consensus on treatment goals intended to optimize psoriasis care by standardizing therapeutic decisions based on endpoints and outcomes measures over defined periods of time [1]. The treatment goal algorithm first originated by Reich and Mrowietz in 2007 [2] and then consented through a Delphi process by a group of experts from 19 European countries has since been adopted into treatment guidelines. They have become an emerging component of routine care. Thus, there is a framework for transforming systematic treatment strategies into daily practice.

Strategies currently recommended for the management of psoriasis tend to be highly technical in nature and regard people with the disease as a homogeneous population, with a similar clinical progression and a similar likelihood of treatment success. However, people with psoriasis represent a heterogeneous population with individual disease expressions

© Springer International Publishing Switzerland 2016
R. Warren and A. Menter (eds.), *Handbook of Psoriasis and Psoriatic Arthritis*, DOI 10.1007/978-3-319-18227-8_5

and personal perceptions about treatment success. For example, Psoriasis Area and Severity Index (PASI)-50-response may be acceptable to one person while others may not rate their treatment as successful until they reach PASI-75-response or PASI-90-response. Similarly, lifestyle considerations are not routinely incorporated into disease management. Taken together, purely clinically driven treatment goals may not be suitable at an individual level and could lead to people not receiving the right treatment at the right time. Therefore, it is necessary that treatment goals and management strategies address the specific needs of the individual as psoriasis frequently requires lifetime control.

As with treatment for rheumatoid arthritis (RA), the systemic treatment of psoriasis thus develops toward an individual but targeted treatment. Since the clinical guidelines mostly refer to data from clinical trials, there is a lack of evidence on the management of psoriasis in particular

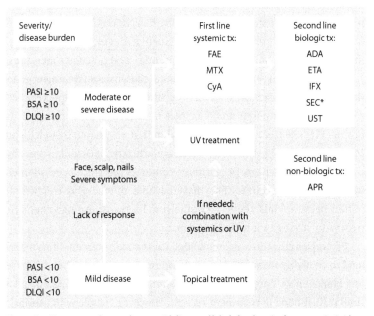

Figure 5.1 Treatment scheme of most guidelines and labels for chronic plaque psoriasis (the order of therapies is alphabetical and does not represent a ranking), adopted from several guidelines for the treatment of moderate-to-severe psoriasis. *First-line status by label. ADA, adalimumab; APR, apremilast; BSA, body surface area; CyA, cyclosporine A; DLQI, Dermatology Life Quality Index; ETA, etanercept; FAE, fumaric acid esters; IFX, infliximab; MTX, methotrexate; PASI, Psoriasis Area and Severity Index; SEC, secukinumab; UST, ustekinumab.

treatment situations which have not yet been subject to clinical trials. These 'challenging treatment situations beyond guidelines' have at least been worked up by expert consensus. As such, an American consensus focused on rare indications and treatments in spite of comorbidities [3–5]. Treatment optimization and transitions were consented by an international expert group, providing expert opinion based on the Delphi consensus [6].

Topical therapy

Topical treatment plays a pivotal role in psoriasis therapy. In mild disease, it is the first treatment of choice and in moderate-to-severe treatment it is used additionally to phototherapy and systemic drugs. There is substantial evidence about the efficacy and safety of the topical drugs [1]. Nevertheless, adherence can be a critical factor, especially in long-term management. It is estimated that 40–50% of patients with psoriasis are non-adherent to topical therapy [7,8]. Adherence in topical treatment is compromised by low- or late-onset of action, often unfavorable galenic characteristics, bad smelling, cosmetic unacceptance, time-consuming application, and low user friendliness. Remarkably, the time needed for treatment is a major predictor for health-related quality of life in psoriasis patients [9]. Taking this into consideration, a low adherence to topical therapy has to be expected. It is thus recommended to choose an effective, well-tolerated and user-friendly long-term product. Shared decision improves long-term adherence. Thus, the crucial points for topical treatment are:

- to involve the patient in the choice of product;
- to explain the need for regular applications;
- to tailor treatment concepts on a long-term basis; and
- to consider proactive treatment regimes in the maintenance phase.

Corticosteroids

First approved in 1952, topical corticosteroids (TCS) are recommended for the treatment of mild-to-severe chronic plaque psoriasis and have become the most prescribed active components [10]. They act via nuclear receptors belonging to the receptor superfamily of retinoid, thyroid, and steroid receptors. As a result of gene expression, but also partly post-transcriptionally, the activity of a number of proteins is modulated in the cell. This leads to a more general modulation of inflammatory reactions, immunosuppression, inhibition of DNA synthesis, and vasoconstriction. The effectiveness of combinations of TCS with calcipotriol, phototherapy, or systemic therapy has been demonstrated, thereby reducing the total dosage of corticosteroids significantly and taking advantage of synergistic effects [10,11]. Choosing the adequate strength and vehicle of administration is important in order to obtain the most benefit with the least potential for side effects. The class of corticosteroids to be prescribed depends on the areas of skin affected. It remains important to be conscious of the possible side effects such as skin atrophy or teleangiectasia, especially when corticosteroids are used as a long-term treatment and are applied in areas prone to these adverse effects (groin, axilla, or under occlusion) [11]. It has been demonstrated that there is no superior effectiveness of twice-daily application over once-daily application, thus it is recommended to start TCS once daily [12,13].

TCS compounds are available in different vehicles, which may also have an impact on the efficacy and potential side effects. Lotions are water-based, weakest in strength, and evaporate. Shampoos may be used for scalp psoriasis but short contact time limits efficacy, making solutions and sprays to be used during the night more effective. Gels are alcohol-based, evaporate quickly, and sting but are equipotent with ointments and solutions. Many patients prefer gels because they are easy to apply and do not disturb clothing. Ointments are petrolatum-based, typically the most potent, and usually do not irritate, making them the best option for sensitive skin. Foams contain alcohol and therefore evaporate quickly, which make them appropriate for application in the hair or for patients (especially men) who prefer this vehicle. Creams are oil in water-based and do not evaporate as quickly but may sting with application. Induction therapy with class III topical steroids is recommended for patients with mild-to-moderate psoriasis vulgaris when not applied to sensitive skin areas [10].

Vitamin D3 analogs (calcipotriol) and calcipotriol/betamethasone

Topical vitamin D3 analogs provide 'steroid-sparing' effects and have a favorable safety profile. Many experts, including a recent consensus conference [11], classify topical vitamin D3 analogs as first-line therapy for psoriasis either as monotherapy or in combination with TCS due to a synergistic, complementary effectiveness. The search strategy identified 21 relevant clinical trials [14]. Best evidence regarding topical long-term treatment was available for the two-compound formulation containing calcipotriene and betamethasone. In comparative trials in psoriasis vulgaris the two-compound formulation showed superior tolerability and cost effectiveness compared with monotherapy [10]. In scalp psoriasis the two-compound gel was superior compared with calcipotriene monotherapy. Standardized and simplified treatment application modes resulted in a better clinical outcome compared with on-demand therapies.

Calcipotriol is started twice daily and then decreased to one to two times daily. Tacalcitol is applied once daily and calcitriol twice daily. The topical treatment should be applied in a thin layer to the affected areas of the skin. For longer term daily use of calcipotriol, no more than 15g should be administered or not more than 100g cream or ointment weekly (maximum body surface area of about 30%). For tacalcitol, the daily maximum is 10g on 15–20% of the body surface area, and for calcitriol 30g ointment daily on up to 35% of the body surface area. Long-term topical treatment with vitamin-D3 analogs in combination with corticosteroids is, according to all available data [15], safe and effective. They may be continued as a maintenance therapy. Best clinical evidence for long-term treatment of psoriasis is available for the two-compound formulation of calcipotriol and betamethasone. In direct comparative trials, the tolerability of (fixed) two-compound formulations was better than the tolerability of vitamin D3 analogs alone [10]. Vitamin D3 analogs are also used in children. Depending on the country, there are different labels with respect to age and maximum body surface to be treated.

Comparative trials on maintenance therapy for psoriasis showed (a) on the body: a trend towards better clinical efficacy of the two-compound formulation compared with the monotherapy with calcipotriol alone; and (b) on the scalp: superior clinical efficacy of the two-compound gel compared with the monotherapy with calcipotriol alone. Patients should be involved in the choice of treatment, formulation, and mode of application. Besides long-term treatment with the two-compound formulation other treatment regimens including calcipotriene monotherapy can also be considered. Due to a favorable risk-benefit ratio in maintenance trials and due to better cost-effectiveness, the application of two-compound products once or twice a week after initial therapy is recommended. In addition to long-term treatment (once to twice weekly) with two-compound formulations, alternative regimens including calcipotriol monotherapy have also been shown to be effective in daily practice [10]. In long-term maintenance, the once-to-twice weekly application of a two-compound formulation is recommended due to its favorable risk-benefit profile and its economic benefits.

Lack of patient adherence leads to suboptimal effectiveness of topical therapy in routine practice. The fixed combination betamethasone/calcipotriol gel is more effective and safer than the administration of single components and may lead to improved patient adherence. Such findings are in line with evidence from randomized controlled trials and a few observational studies demonstrating superior clinical outcomes, quality of life, tolerability, and lower risk of side effect in patients treated with the fixed combination of betamethasone/calcipotriol gel [16].

Coal tar

Coal tar is included in antipsoriatics, antiseptics, and antipruriginous preparations. The acceptance of coal tar preparations is low due to their color and odor. The availability of more practical and effective alternatives has reduced the use of coal tar as monotherapy for plaque psoriasis. Only when therapeutically necessary, coal tar or pix lithanthracis may be used alone or in combination with ultraviolet B (UVB) or psoralen ultraviolet A (PUVA) to treat recalcitrant chronic plaque psoriasis. Coal tar has mainly been used in psoriasis to increase the effectiveness of subsequent UV light therapy. Therapy was often based on the 'Goeckermann scheme', which includes a tar-based topical therapy, followed by UVB (suberythematous dose) after removing the preparation. Erythema, if it occurs, may be a helpful guide for adjusting the dosage. However, there is general consensus that long-term therapy is not recommended. There is still controversy about the potential of a carcinogenic effect resulting in squamous cell cancer, although data from patient registries or clinical studies have failed to provide concise evidence. Clinical studies on coal tar with phototherapy have reported mixed results. Studies report that after 15 to 20 treatments with UV therapy, 45–80% of patients achieve at least PASI-75 [10]. However, the additive effect of coal tar, compared with UV therapy alone, has not been sufficiently proven.

Dithranol

Until the early 1980s dithranol (1,8-dihydroxy-9-anthrone; synonyms: anthralin and cignolin) was the most common topical therapy for psoriasis vulgaris in Europe. Newer topical therapies (steroids and vitamin D3 derivatives) have replaced dithranol, especially in outpatient care since the irritative effects and prolonged skin discoloration was a common reason for discomfort and patient dissatisfaction. Dithranol suppresses cell proliferation in vitro and in vivo. It also inhibits neutrophilic granulocytes and monocytes, the migration of leukocytes, and lymphocyte proliferation. Finally, it has also strong antiproliferative effects on keratinocytes due to the inhibition of the epidermal growth factor (EGF) receptor and binding of the ligand to the EGF receptor, in addition to the inhibition of necessary signaling cascades by protein tyrosine kinase (PTK). There is also evidence for inhibition of the proinflammatory cytokines interleukin (IL)-6 and IL-8 from monocytes, possibly due to a DNA-inhibiting effect [17].

Dithranol/anthralin monotherapy is recommended in patients with moderate-to-severe psoriasis for induction therapy during hospitalization or outpatient treatment under close meshed guidance [10]. 'Classic' dithranol therapy treatment of plaques is launched with the lowest concentration (0.1% or less), applying a thin layer of the drug once daily. The ointment should not be removed. The concentration is gradually increased, depending on the level of irritation and patient discomfort. The target concentration is 1–3%. In case of severe skin irritation, dosage may be reduced temporarily. Dithranol short-contact therapy may be an alternative treatment to phototherapy or systemic therapy in patients with moderate-to-severe psoriasis. Within this treatment modality 1% cream is applied for 10 minutes during the first few days of therapy and then removed with tepid water. The length of application (for either drug) is then gradually increased to 30 minutes over the following days. Dithranol ointment is then increased to 1, 2, or 3% concentration. It should be applied if possible for 10–20 minutes for 3–4 days at each time.

In patients who do not respond or have a contraindication to calcipotriol, corticosteroids, photo(chemo)therapy, systemic therapy, and biologics, dithranol may be a safe alternative. Treatment duration should not exceed 4–8 weeks, and 2–3 weeks of therapy are usually necessary before there is any notable improvement. There are no reports of rebound effects after stopping therapy. Maintenance or long-term therapy is impractical and has no advantages. Given the higher efficacy in treating severe chronic plaque-type psoriasis, it is recommended to add phototherapy or topical preparations (vitamin D3 analogs and corticosteroids) to dithranol treatment [10]. However, treatment is limited by irritation, especially of the normal skin surrounding the treatment area, thus it is suitable only for large plaques. A barrier cream can be used to 'mask' around the area for treatment. In an outpatient setting, dithranol is usually used as 'short-contact therapy'. The results of clinical studies, some of them being methodically acceptable, show total remission (PASI reduction of 100%) in 30–70% and partial remission (PASI reduction of 75%) in 26–100% of patients after 5–8 weeks [10]. The safety of the drug is uncontested. Burning, redness, and transitory brown discoloration are the only adverse effects reported. There are no reports of adverse systemic effects.

Vitamin A (tazarotene)

Tazarotene, being a potent third-generation retinoid, has been available as tazarotene gel 0.05% and 0.1% for the treatment of mild-to-moderate psoriasis vulgaris. Tazarotene is hydrolyzed in the skin by esterases to form its active metabolite, tazarotenic acid, binding to the nuclear retinoic acid receptors (RAR)-beta and RAR-gamma and thus affecting differentiation and epidermal proliferation. It leads to a reduced expression of inflammatory mediators in the epidermis and dermis. Tazarotene gel 0.1% is applied in a thin film once per day (in the evenings) to the affected sites (no more than 10% of the body surface area). The drug should be applied directly to the lesion, avoiding contact with healthy skin or skin folds given its irritative effects. After 12 weeks of treatment with tazarotene 0.1% once daily about 50% of patients achieve at least a 50% improvement in skin lesions [18]. Given its potentially irritative effects on the skin, tazarotene is often combined with topical steroids. Commonly reported side effects include itching, burning, and redness at the application site. There are no reports of phototoxic or photoallergic reactions. Patients should avoid excessive UV light exposure and should wear protective clothing against sunlight during therapy. The use of tazarotene may be considered in the treatment of localized mild-to-moderate psoriasis vulgaris although topicals containing tazarotene are not available in many countries.

Calcineurin inhibitors

The topical calcineurin inhibitors tacrolimus and pimecrolimus reduce the action of calcineurin, a protein phosphatase involved in activating T-cells. They are a potential alternative to TCS because of their ability to suppress T-cell activation and proliferation. By blocking calcineurin phosphatase, they prevent the dephosphorylation of the nuclear factor of activated T cells, which leads to inhibition of T-cell activation and the consecutive production of proinflammatory cytokines (tumor necrosis factor α [TNF-α], interferon γ [IFN-γ], and IL-2 being key cytokines in the activation and amplification of T-cell response) [19]. Topical calcineurin inhibitors are approved for the treatment of atopic dermatitis. Their use in psoriasis vulgaris is based on the results from clinical studies which, however, have not led to approval by US FDA or EMA. The efficacy can be compared to that of class II corticosteroids. Out of eight studies on topical calcineurin inhibitors (pimecrolimus, tacrolimus) for psoriasis, four studies reported a significant improvement or complete clearance of lesions in 40–50% of patients after six to twelve weeks [10].

Tacrolimus and pimecrolimus may be used once to twice daily for chronic plaque-type psoriasis in the face, flexures, and anogenital region as an additive (interval treatment) or as a replacement of corticosteroids [10]. Brief pre-therapy with topical steroids is often advised. The use on other locations is not recommended not least because of the off-label status and higher costs. Application may be of benefit until clearance of psoriatic lesions is reached and should be followed by regular skin care (ie, basic treatment and ointments without active components). Tacrolimus is available as an ointment in concentrations of 0.03% and 0.1%. Pimecrolimus 1% is available as a cream. Both components do not induce skin atrophy and there has been no evidence of substantial systemic absorption.

Phototherapy

Various ultraviolet B (UVB) and ultraviolet A (UVA) wavelengths may be used for the treatment of psoriasis vulgaris. Phototherapy triggers various biological effects that may contribute to its anti-psoriatic effects. These include anti-inflammatory action, such as reduced mobility of antigen-presenting Langerhans cells, inhibition of T-lymphocyte activation, and the induction of programmed cell death (apoptosis) of activated T-lymphocytes. Furthermore, epidermal hyperproliferation is inhibited by interactions with keratinocyte DNA, as psoralen plus ultraviolet A (PUVA) also interferes with DNA synthesis. There are also potentially relevant anti-angiogenic effects, that have not been elucidated yet. UVB and PUVA are recommended for induction therapy for moderate-to-severe psoriasis vulgaris, especially in patients with a large body surface area involved and relevant contraindications towards systemic treatment options [10]. Caution is needed in patients with skin types I and II as well as in any condition of UV sensitivity, including uptake of sensitizing drugs.

UV maintenance therapy is not recommended owing to decreased efficacy after repetitive UV-exposure and increased chance of UV skin damage. A limitation of treatment courses to a maximum of two per year has been recommended, although concise evidence on the long-term therapy is lacking. UV-therapy after or during immunosuppressant medication, especially cyclosporine, requires profound attention. Performing phototherapy requires comprehensive clinical experience on the part of the physician. Given the number of variables involved, there is a wide array of treatment protocols that the physician has to be acquainted with.

UVB therapy
Originally, broadband UVB light with wavelengths of 280–315 nm was used for treatment of psoriasis. Since the 1980s, however, phototherapy has increasingly focused on using a narrower spectrum.

Broadband ultraviolet B
Studies on broadband UVB reported the results of two, three, five, and seven exposures weekly. The proportion of patients who achieved a PASI-75 improvement varied among different studies. The majority of studies reported a PASI-75 response in 50–75% of patients [20–28]. The amount of time needed to achieve this level of improvement decreased with increasing number of exposures.

Selective UV therapy
Studies on selective UV (SUV) therapy investigated the effectiveness of three exposures per week or once daily [29–37]. A PASI-75 improvement or better was achieved in 29% of patients treated three times weekly and in 86% who were treated daily (within 4 weeks in this group). The latter study also directly compared SUP with broadband UVB therapy and found SUP to be more effective.

Long-term use of UVB phototherapy may result in sun damage and premature aging of the skin. Controversy exists about the maximum dose to avoid potential carcinogenic effects of UVB phototherapy. There are still only insufficient data available on the use of UVB therapy in humans, therefore recommendations could not be provided for long-term treatment.

Psoralen ultraviolet A therapy
Photochemotherapy combines topical application or systemic administration of a photosensitizer followed by phototherapy with the appropriate

wavelength, usually UVA. Since the 1970s, the administration of photosensitizing psoralens followed by whole-body or partial-body UVA phototherapy (315–400 nm), has been supported by scientific findings.

Psoralens may be given systemically, as oral PUVA therapy, or topically as a bath or cream. Treatments should be administered in specialized centers providing sufficient expertise and awareness of the risk-benefit ratio. Before beginning oral PUVA therapy, the patient should be examined by an ophthalmologist and protective goggles should be obtained together with comprehensive education on the conduction during therapy.

High-dose phototherapy is associated with increased risk of burning, and long-term use is associated with increased skin cancer risk, especially with UVA. Some investigators recommend limiting lifetime PUVA treatments to fewer than 200 sessions although data are insufficient regarding the maximum number of phototherapy sessions allowable for patients with darker skin types.

The carcinogenic effects associated with an increased risk of developing spinocellular and basal cell cancer depending on cumulative UVA dose are well established. Although there are reports on an increased risk of melanoma following long-term therapy, the actual risk is still unclear. Oral PUVA therapy can also lead to disorders of pigmentation, brown spots (PUVA lentigines), and cataracts. The treating physician should conduct a thorough inspection of the entire body surface, especially for signs of cancerous lesions, precancerous lesions, and dysplastic nevus cell nevi. The patient should be informed about the course of therapy, possible side effects, and potential long-term risks. Synergistic effects resulting from additional UV exposure during leisure time or self-treatment have also to be taken into consideration.

The UV dose must be precisely recorded (J/cm^2 or mJ/cm^2). Erythema development must be controlled regularly before increasing the dosage. Regular monitoring of therapy includes documentation of treatment outcomes, side effects, and any concomitant therapy use. Unless they are the focus of therapy, chronic sun-exposed areas (face,neck and backs of the hands) and genital regions should be protected from exposure to UV light. Adequate protective measures against exposure to sunlight are necessary during therapy. After completing a treatment series, the cumulative UV dosage and the number of treatment sessions must be recorded and given to the patient. Patients with a high cumulative UV dose should undergo lifelong regular skin cancer screening. Despite the superior efficacy of PUVA compared with UVB therapy alone, narrow band UVB therapy may be considered as the first choice for phototherapy. Given the availability of targeted systemic treatment options and taking the related comorbidities into consideration, phototherapy remains a treatment option for preselected patients.

Systemic therapy

Systemic therapies are recommended for patients with moderate-to-severe disease or when adequate control of disease cannot be achieved with topical agents. The indication for systemic therapy, including biologics, needs to be based on the clinical severity and previous treatments as well as on patient factors including quality of life, patient preferences, and patient compliance (Figure 5.2). Moreover, comorbidities need to be taken into account for the following reasons:

- the comorbidity can be a potential co-target of treatment, eg, arthritis;
- the comorbidity can have an impact on treatment response, eg, obesity;
- the comorbidity can be a contraindication for treatment, eg, liver disease in methotrexate (MTX) treatment;
- the comorbidity may increase the risk for side effects; and
- drugs for the treatment of the comorbidity may interfere with systemic psoriasis treatment.

There is a variety of systemic drugs available. Optimized treatment choice includes the assessment of safety/tolerability for induction or maintenance therapy, as well as the feasibility of therapy for the doctor and patient, patient defined needs, costs/benefits aspects and country-dependent regulations (Figure 5.1). The data from international pharmacoeconomic studies are not entirely applicable to the situation in every country given differences between the systems and regulations of reimbursement.

	Indication for systemic therapy		
Clinical criteria	**Drug profile**	**Patient characteristics**	**Label & legal**
Psoriasis phenotype & locations	Effectiveness on psoriasis & psoriatic arthritis	Preferences	Label
Severity	Effectiveness on comorbidity	Age, gender	Costs
Comorbidity	Safety	Socio-economics	Regulations
Pre-treatments	Feasibility	Adherence	Availability

Figure 5.2 Considerations for selecting systemic drugs in psoriasis. Reproduced with permission from © M Augustin, 2015.

Methotrexate

MTX has been a mainstay of psoriasis treatment for decades. It shows anti-inflammatory, antiproliferative, and immunosuppressant characteristics. The main mode of action is the competitive inhibition of the enzyme dihydrofolate reductase, thus acting as a folic acid antagonist. Because it received regulatory approval before carefully conducted clinical trials were required, evidence-based protocols for psoriasis treatment are rare. There is still no comparative study directly addressing the therapeutic strategies (ie, the questions of starting dose, method of escalation, and route of administration) for MTX in psoriasis. Data from health research studies reveal a marked variability among dermatologists in how MTX is administered and monitored [38].

According to the different guidelines [39] for MTX in the treatment of psoriasis vulgaris, weekly doses of MTX (up to 25 mg) can be administered through oral or parenteral (intramuscular or subcutaneous) routes in a single dose. Although subcutaneous injection of MTX increases the therapeutic efficiency and decreases the risk of gastrointestinal side effects, there is still not enough evidence relating to psoriasis vulgaris. There is no general agreement about the starting dose of MTX; some physicians generally start with low doses (eg, 7.5 mg/week) and gradually increase, whereas others recommend starting at the anticipated target dose (eg, 15 mg/week). Injection therapy is preferable due to individually variable bioavailability of orally administered MTX and better tolerability.

In any case, the dosage should be adjusted based on the response, individual tolerance and patient needs. Treatment studies reveal that adequate therapeutic response is achieved gradually within the first 12–16 weeks following start of treatment, and MTX has a dose-dependent effect. After 16 weeks of treatment with MTX 25–50% of patients achieve a reduction in PASI of 75% [10]. The maximum efficacy of MTX is not reached until after the induction phase, regardless of dosing scheme. MTX is suitable for long-term therapy, always monitoring safety and tolerability [6].

Based on currently available evidence, folic acid supplementation may reduce hematologic, mucocutaneous, and gastrointestinal adverse effects (especially liver toxicity) of MTX, but may also slightly impair MTX efficacy in psoriasis [38]. Folate supplementation for patients with folate deficiency or those who have high needs of folate (eg, during some infectious diseases or certain antibiotic therapy) and in patients being treated with high-dose MTX is universally accepted, but there is no general consensus on the need for folic acid or folinic acid supplementation [40]. Based on the recommendations by a panel of European dermatologists [41], prescription of folic acid supplementation with MTX therapy is recommended at a dose of 5 mg/d for 1–3 days, to be taken 24–48 hours after the MTX dose.

There is no indication for liver biopsy before and during MTX treatment except in rare cases of liver disease. However, pre-screening for MTX treatment includes the assessment of risks for severe liver damage, serum levels of amino-terminal propeptide type III procollagen (PIIINP), and liver function tests (LFT). It should be noted that test reliability may be reduced by factors such as smoking, taking non-steroidal anti-inflammatory drugs (NSAIDs), or other drugs as well as joint involvement and general systemic inflammation. Pre-treatment procedures also include chest X-ray (in case of any pulmonary infections during therapy) and careful patient selection and informed consent. It is crucial to inform the patient on how to take the drug (only once weekly) and about early symptoms of potential adverse effects.

During therapy, strict monitoring, use of the lowest possible effective dose (maximum 25 mg/week), and additional use of folic acid or folinic acid allows for an acceptable safety profile. The importance of strict contraception for at least three months after therapy (men and women) has to be communicated to the patient. MTX is suitable for use with TNF-α inhibitors. MTX may also be used in patients with concomitant PsA. Of all systemic antipsoriatic agents, MTX has the lowest medication costs per day [10].

Under MTX treatment liver disease may occur. Moreover, myelosuppression has been reported, especially in patients with kidney insufficiency. As with other potential side effects, acute pneumonitis and alveolitis are uncommon but have to be communicated to the patient as potential serious adverse events. To date, the former recommended cumulative life-time dose of 1.5g MTX is now considered as a guide. If long-term treatment does not induce any abnormalities and is well-tolerated, longer treatment periods with higher cumulative dose may be considered.

Cyclosporine A

Since the early 1990s, cyclosporine A has become an established treatment choice for psoriasis. It is approved for moderate-to-severe psoriasis for patients eligible for systemic treatment. Due to its inhibiting effect on immune functions, especially in T cells, cyclosporine is considered a selective immunosuppressant.

The availability of cyclosporine (peak concentration, clearance of oral cyclosporine) depends primarily on the activity of the intestinal transporter protein P-glycoprotein (PGp) and hepatic activity of the 3A family of the cytochrome P450 system (CYP3A family). The expression of PGp can vary due to genetic factors and CYP3A4 activity also exhibits up to a 50-fold variability in the general population. In addition, the CYP3A family is responsible for Phase I biotransformation of a large group of medications, many of which are substrates or modulators of CYP3A or PGp, and may thus potentially influence the breakdown of cyclosporine.

Because cyclosporine has a narrow therapeutic spectrum, knowledge of possible interactions is crucial for all physicians who treat patients with cyclosporine or who plan to use it.

For treatment initiation, a dosage of 2.5–3 mg/kg of body weight is standard. A study [42] on dosages based on weight (1.25–5 mg/kg of body weight per day) compared with dosages that were independent of body weight (100–300 mg/daily) reported that a strict weight-adjusted dosing was superior. The daily dose is generally divided in half and taken mornings and evenings. The microemulsion should be taken before meals. If there is an inadequate response to the initial dosage of 2.5–3 mg/kg of body weight after 4–6 weeks, the dose may be increased to a maximum of 5 mg/kg of body weight. If after another 4–6 weeks, healing is still insufficient, cyclosporine should be discontinued. For patients with severe disease in whom a more rapid effect is desired, treatment may begin with an initial dosage of 5 mg/kg of body weight.

Cyclosporine is recommended for induction therapy of patients with moderate-to-severe psoriasis [10]. For long-term therapy, after 1–2 years maximum, discontinuation of therapy should be considered due to potential long-term side effects, especially nephrotoxicity, hypertension, and the increased risk of cancer. Given the large number of patients who have been treated with cyclosporine (for other diseases as well), the risk profile of undesirable adverse effects is well-known.

Drug interactions need to be observed carefully, on the one hand because of altered availability of cyclosporine or the concomitant drug and on the other hand because of an increased risk of adverse effects. Combination use with topical preparations is helpful in the treatment of plaque psoriasis, especially as it appears that concomitant local therapy with vitamin D3 analogs or steroids can help reduce cyclosporine dosage without diminishing its effectiveness and may reduce the time to achieve treatment response, especially during the induction phase. As is the case with other immunosuppressant drugs, cyclosporine is associated with an increased risk of lymphoproliferative disorders and other malignant tumors, especially skin tumors. Patients with psoriasis vulgaris who have received numerous phototherapy treatments (especially higher cumulative dosages of PUVA, eg, >1.000 J/cm^2) have an increased risk of skin cancer, in particular squamous cell carcinoma.

Acitretin

Acitretin is a traditional systemic treatment for psoriasis with antiproliferative and immunomodulatory properties [43]. The retinoids were first synthesized in the 1970s to assess their usefulness in skin cancer, and their use in dermatology was soon extended to the treatment of other proliferative diseases. In psoriasis, their usefulness arises from their effects on keratinization, cell proliferation and inflammation, and immune regulation [44]. Acitretin acts, at least in part, by inhibiting interleukin 6–driven induction of helper T cells (subtype 17), which has a major role in the pathogenesis of psoriasis [5]. Acitretin may have an added effectiveness when combined with a biologic (although off-label in combination) and could be considered in patients for whom immunosuppression is not desirable. As with all the synthetic retinoids, acitretin is highly teratogenic, and this risk – further increased by the drug's long elimination half-life – greatly restricts its use in women of reproductive potential.

The recommended starting dosage for acitretin in plaque psoriasis is 10–20 mg/d. This initial regimen should be continued for 4 weeks. Response to treatment should be assessed at 4 weeks, after which the dose should be gradually increased to achieve the best therapeutic effect with the fewest adverse effects (minimal effective dose). In general, the maintenance regimen varies between 25–50 mg/d. Psoriatic lesions clear faster when the starting dose is higher, but such high-dose regimens also increase the risk of mucocutaneous adverse effects and consequently the risk of the patient stopping treatment due to poor tolerance of side effects. Initiating treatment at a high dosage (1 mg/kg/d) is currently only recommended for the treatment of generalized flares of pustular psoriasis. It usually takes 3–6 months to achieve maximum response. The effectiveness of low-dose retinoids as monotherapy in moderate-to-severe psoriasis vulgaris is not satisfactory.

After 8–12 weeks, at a dosage of 0.4 mg/kg of body weight to maximum 40 mg/daily, 23–30% of patients achieve PASI-75 [10]. Although the drug is more effective at higher dosages, the related side effects are also often greater, with involvement of the skin and mucous membranes. One advantage of retinoids is their synergistic effects when used in combination with UV phototherapy [10]. In some patients, psoriasis may worsen after the start of treatment, a phenomenon that manifests as more intense erythema and a greater spread of lesions, which later resolve. For long-term therapy, ossification has to be excluded by radiologic examination of the spine and joints. Women of childbearing age must ensure effective contraception for up to 2 years after therapy and patients have to be advised not to donate blood at any time during treatment and up to 1 year after.

Apremilast

Agents that increase intracellular cyclic adenosine monophosphate reduce the production of proinflammatory mediators, such as TNF-α, IL-23, and interferon. Inhibitors selective for phosphodiesterase 4 have been shown to improve inflammation in psoriasis. Apremilast, an oral small molecule inhibitor of phosphodiesterase 4, has been investigated extensively for psoriasis, ankylosing spondylitis, Behçet's syndrome, atopic dermatitis, and rheumatoid arthritis. Apremilast was studied in patients with moderate-to-severe psoriasis in a Phase III study [45] where 33% of patients achieved a PASI-75 at week 16 compared with 5% in the placebo arm.

The advantages of apremilast include its oral administration, acceptable tolerability and safety, growing experience in patients with PsA, and an extensive study program. Given the lower PASI response rate compared to other agents, the target patient group that best suits this treatment approach has to be tailored in everyday practice and evaluated by patient registries and a concise postmarketing surveillance program. Apremilast has been approved by the US FDA for PsA and EMA for moderate-to-severe plaque-type psoriasis in adult patients who failed to respond to, have a contraindication to, or who are intolerant to other systemic therapy such as cyclosporine, methotrexate, or PUVA.

Biologics

Although phototherapy and conventional systemic agents are effective for some patients, others experience inadequate response or marked side effects. In recent years, major advances in our understanding of the pathogenesis of psoriasis have facilitated the development of highly selective biologic agents that revolutionized modern psoriasis treatment. Etanercept, adalimumab, infliximab, and ustekinumab, have been implemented consecutively for moderate-to-severe psoriasis. For PsA, these agents, as well as golimumab and certolizumab, have been introduced into the markets. In addition, secukinumab has recently been introduced into clinical practice.

In plaque-type psoriasis without arthritis, the TNF-α antagonists and ustekinumab are generally indicated for adult patients who failed to respond to, who have a contraindication to, or who are intolerant to therapies such as cyclosporine, methotrexate, PUVA therapy or narrowband UVB. By contrast, according to the EMA label, secukinumab is indicated for moderate-to-severe plaque-type psoriasis 'in adults who are candidates for systemic therapy', thus providing a 'first-line' status similar to the other conventional systemic drugs. All biologics have been shown to be highly effective even when conventional systemic treatments have failed (Table 5.1).

The systemic treatment of psoriasis with biologics is in general divided into two phases: induction and maintenance. Typically, the induction

	PASI-50, % (95% CI)	PASI-75, % (95% CI)	PASI-90, % (95% CI)
Adalimumab	81 (74–87)	58 (49–68)	30 (23–39)
Etanercept 25 mg 2 x wk	65 (56–73)	39 (30–48)	15 (10–21)
Etanercept 50 mg 2 x wk	76 (71–81)	52 (45–59)	24 (19–30)
Infliximab	93 (89–96)	80 (70–87)	54 (42–64)
Placebo	13 (12–14)	4 (3–4)	1 (0–1)
Ustekinumab[a] 45 mg	88 (84–91)	69 (62–75)	40 (33–48)
Ustekinumab[a] 90 mg	90 (87–93)	74 (68–80)	46 (39–54)

Table 5.1 Comparative efficacy of biologics for the management of plaque-type psoriasis across trials in the induction phase. [a]Ustekinumab data are taken from clinical trials in which the doses used were not those specified in the current summary of product characteristics; however, the data used in this meta-analysis relate to weight-adjusted doses. PASI, Psoriasis Area and Severity. Reproduced with permission from © John Wiley & Sons, 2012. All rights reserved. Reich et al [46].

phase comprises the first 12–16 weeks although, depending on the drug and dosage, it may be prolonged to 24 weeks. Maintenance therapy is started once induction is complete, and a PASI reduction of at least 50% or other relevant benefits is achieved. The regimen prescribed must take into account the particular characteristics of long-term biologic treatment.

Definition of treatment failure is a consideration of great importance in biologic therapy because it generally requires a change of biologic agent and increases the cost of treatment. Primary treatment failure is defined as the failure during the induction phase to obtain a 50% improvement in PASI from baseline (PASI 50) known as the efficacy threshold. Although the lack of a PASI-50 response is the key criterion for treatment failure in the formulation of treatment goals, the decision has to be taken on a case-by-case basis taking patients' needs into account. Secondary treatment failure is defined as loss of the PASI-50 response during the maintenance phase, although other definitions can be established based on an absolute PASI score, the physician global assessment (PGA), or a combination of PASI and a quality-of-life score.

Etanercept

Etanercept is a human TNF receptor (p75) Fc fusion protein. Its terminal elimination half-life is about 4–5 days. As a soluble receptor, etanercept binds free TNF-α and has been used successfully in the treatment of RA, PsA, and other forms of arthritis [47,48]. Etanercept is also an effective treatment option in psoriasis [49–51] and is approved for the treatment of adult patients with moderate-to-severe psoriasis vulgaris (plaque psoriasis) in whom other systemic therapies including cyclosporine, MTX, and PUVA have failed, are contraindicated, or are not tolerated. The recommended adult dosage for the treatment of plaque psoriasis is 25 mg twice weekly or 50 mg once weekly (Table 5.2).

If there is high disease activity, or the patient is overweight, an initial dose of 50 mg twice weekly may be given for up to 12 weeks, followed by 25 mg twice weekly or 50 mg once weekly. Doses of 50 mg once weekly have become the most practicable and favorable treatment regime. In the European Union, etanercept is also approved for use in patients from the age of six years with long-term severe plaque psoriasis.

	Etanercept	Infliximab	Adalimumab	Ustekinumab
Approx. elimination half-life	4 d	9 d	15 d	21 d
Dosage regimens	50 mg sc 1 x wk or 25 mg 2 x wk for up to 24 wks, or 50 mg 2 x wk for the first 12 wks. Continuous therapy is appropriate for some adult patients	Induction regimen of 5 mg/wk iv wks 0, 2, and 6 and every 8 wks thereafter	First dose 80 mg sc, 40 mg after 1 wk and then 40 mg every 2 wks thereafter	First dose of 45 mg sc, followed by 45 mg 4 wks later and then 45 mg every 12 wks thereafter. (In patients weighing >100 kg, doses are doubled). The 45 mg dose has also been shown to be effective. However, efficacy is greater with the 90 mg dose
Onset of clinical effect usually occurs within:	4–8 wks	1–2 wks	2–4 wks	2–4 wks
Main risks[a]	Tuberculosis and other infections; rheumatologic registers show a lower risk of tuberculosis and serious infections than with anti-TNF antibodies	Tuberculosis and other infections	Tuberculosis and other infections	Tuberculosis and other infections. The SPC includes no special considerations relating to patients with heart failure, demyelinating disease, or autoimmune disease in contrast to those cited in the case of anti-TNF antibodies
Special observations	Approved in the EU for use in pediatric patients aged ≥6 yrs, 0.8 mg/kg (max 50 mg per dose) 1 x wk for 24 wks max. Approved for psoriatic arthritis	Approved for psoriatic arthritis	Approved for psoriatic arthritis	Effective in psoriatic arthritis, but not approved for this indication

Table 5.2 Characteristics of biologics for the management of plaque-type psoriasis. [a]Vaccines with live or attenuated germs (varicella, zoster, or yellow fever in adults) are contraindicated in all these patients. iv, intravenous; sc, subcutaneous; SPC, summary of product characteristics. Reproduced with permission from © John Wiley & Sons, 2012. All rights reserved. Reich et al [46].

The maximum efficacy of etanercept is not reached until after the induction phase. Etanercept is suitable for long-term use. Based on the data from published studies, an increase in effectiveness in long-term therapy of psoriasis vulgaris may be expected in some patients. The efficacy and safety of etanercept are not influenced by the development of antibodies to the drug, as they do not seem to be neutralizing. Various safety aspects should be considered when administering etanercept. One of the most important is the risk of infection. Given the widespread use of etanercept (for other diseases as well), the risk of side effects related to its use is readily assessed. Combination use of etanercept with MTX can have synergistic effects, especially in patients with a slow response during induction phase [52].

Adalimumab

Adalimumab binds with high affinity and specificity to soluble and membrane-bound TNF-α. This prevents binding to the TNF-α-receptor (p55 and p75) and blocks the biologic effect of TNF-α. Based on results from two pivotal Phase III trials [53,54], adalimumab is approved for use in adults with moderate-to-severe plaque psoriasis who did not tolerate or failed to respond to systemic therapies including MTX, cyclosporine, and PUVA therapy, or who have contraindications to these treatments (for indications for PsA see Chapter 6). It is furthermore approved in the EU for the treatment of severe chronic plaque psoriasis in children and adolescents from 4 years of age who have had an inadequate response to or are inappropriate candidates for topical therapy and phototherapies. The usual adult dose for subcutaneous (sc) injection is 80 mg of adalimumab at week 0 (initial administration), followed by 40 mg after 1 week, and every 2 weeks from week 3. The effect of adalimumab is usually obtained within 4–16 weeks after the initiation of treatment. If the effect is not obtained within 16 weeks (failure to achieve PASI-50), the continuation of the treatment should be considered carefully, including the combination therapy with MTX. During the induction phase, adalimumab is one of the most effective medications for the treatment of psoriasis vulgaris and it is suitable for long-term therapy. In patients with concomitant PsA, administration of TNF-α antagonists is especially useful. The safety profile is comparable to other TNF-α antagonists approved for psoriasis, although half-life differs from etanercept and has to be considered when discontinuing therapy due to safety reasons.

Ustekinumab

Ustekinumab is a recombinant human IgG1 antibody. It binds with high specificity and affinity to the common p40 subunit of the cytokines IL-12 and IL-23, which prevents their interaction with the IL-12Rß1 receptor on nature killer cells and T lymphocytes. This in turn impairs the IL-12 and IL-23 signaling-dependent maturation and expansion of Th1 and Th17 cells. At 20 days the terminal elimination half time is about the same as natural IgG1.

Ustekinumab is approved for use in the treatment of moderate-to-severe psoriasis vulgaris in adult patients who did not respond to other systemic therapies including cyclosporine A, MTX, and PUVA, or in whom these are contraindicated or not tolerated (for PsA indications see Chapter 6). Ustekinumab was more effective than placebo or etanercept in three randomized, double-blind, multicentre phase III trials in adult patients with moderate to severe plaque psoriasis. PHOENIX 1 [55] and PHOENIX 2 [56] were placebo-controlled trials, and the ACCEPT trial was an active comparator trial against etanercept [57]. In all three trials, ustekinumab 45 mg or 90 mg significantly improved clinical symptoms of psoriasis compared with placebo or etanercept. Since 2015, ustekinumab has been approved in the EU for the treatment of moderate-to-severe plaque psoriasis in adolescent patients from the age of 12 years and older, who are inadequately controlled by, or are intolerant to, other systemic therapies or phototherapies.

In patients weighing less than 100 kg, 45 mg of ustekinumab sc is injected at week 0 (initial administration) and at week 4, followed by 12-week intervals. If the patient shows inadequate response, the dose can be increased to 90 mg. In patients weighing over 100 kg the starting dose is 90 mg per injection. When the treatment effect of ustekinumab is not obtained within 24 weeks of the initiation of administration, modification of treatment plan, including the dose increase from 45 to 90 mg, should be considered on an individual basis. Ustekinumab is suitable for long-term therapy.

Infliximab

Infliximab binds specifically to soluble, transmembranous and receptor-bound TNF-α. Binding blocks soluble TNF-α and its proinflammatory activity is neutralized. Binding to membrane cell-bound TNF-α causes elimination of affected cells, possibly as a result of complement activation and/or antibody-dependent cellular cytotoxicity, or due to induction of apoptosis.

Infliximab is efficacious as induction and maintenance therapy in the treatment of moderate-to-severe plaque psoriasis in the pivotal Phase III EXPRESS and EXPRESS II trials [58,59]. Infliximab is indicated for treatment of moderate-to-severe plaque psoriasis in adult patients who failed to respond to, have a contraindication to, or are intolerant to other systemic therapy including cyclosporine, MTX, or PUVA. Infliximab, at 5 mg/kg bodyweight, is intravenously (IV) infused slowly over 2 hours or longer on constant observation of the administrating physician. The drug is infused at 2 and 6 weeks after the initial infusion, followed by every 8 weeks. At week 14 and after, 1 hour infusion is allowed only if no infusion reactions occur throughout the first three infusions and the physician is acquainted with the review on the management of infusion reactions. The dose can be adjusted according to bodyweight because infliximab is administrated IV at a dose of 5 mg/kg of bodyweight. Unlike in the treatment of RA, however, the dose escalation or shortening of treatment intervals due to the decreased effect is currently not recommended in the treatment of psoriasis. Acute infusion reactions are a commonly reported side effect of infliximab. Usually these reactions are mild with chills, headache, flush, nausea, dyspnea, or infiltration at the infusion site. The probability of an infusion reaction is increased in patients with infliximab-specific antibodies. Anaphylactoid reactions, irrespective of infliximab-specific antibodies, are also possible. Thus patient monitoring with the possibility of emergency care during infusion and for 1 hour afterward is required. Especially after a long treatment-free interval, renewed treatment initiation may lead to arthralgia, myalgia, Quincke edema, or other acute reactions.

Several safety aspects must be taken into consideration for the use of infliximab. The most important are infusion reactions and the risk of serious infection. This requires a careful assessment of the indications for its use, and thorough education and monitoring of the patient. Therapy should be given continuously every eight weeks in order to prevent more frequent infusion reactions as can occur with episodic administration. Combination therapy with infliximab and MTX may help prevent the formation of antibodies, although data on the exact mechanism and the appropriate dosing of MTX are lacking.

Secukinumab

In the environment of systemic inflammation and especially psoriasis, IL-17 has several key activities. IL-17 recruits TH17 cells and myeloid dendritic cells, promotes neutrophil migration, and increases antimicrobial peptides enhancing innate immunity. Furthermore, IL-17 stimulates angiogenesis and vascular inflammation associated with atherosclerosis, a possible milestone to cardiovascular risk in patients with psoriasis. Six isoforms of IL-17 have been identified (IL-17A, B, C, D, F, and γ). With respect to psoriasis, IL-17A is highly expressed in skin lesions and has become a target of therapeutic development. Emerging evidence suggests a central role of IL-17 and IL-23/T17 axis in the pathogenesis of psoriasis, giving a rationale for using IL-17-blocking agents as therapeutics [60].

Secukinumab is a recombinant, high-affinity, fully human monoclonal antibody that selectively binds and neutralizes interleukin-17A. It has been evaluated in Phase III trials, including two pivotal trials, known as ERASURE (Efficacy of Response and Safety of 2 Fixed Secukinumab Regimens in Psoriasis) and FIXTURE (Safety and Efficacy of Secukinumab Compared to Etanercept in Subjects With Moderate-to-Severe, Chronic Plaque-Type Psoriasis) [61]. In the randomized, placebo-controlled ERASURE trial involving 738 patients with moderate or severe plaque psoriasis, patients received secukinumab 300 mg or 150 mg or placebo, administered once a week for 4 weeks and then every 4 weeks thereafter. Placebo-treated patients who did not achieve PASI-75 responses after 12 weeks were randomized consecutively to 300 mg or 150 mg of secukinumab. Therapy was maintained in all groups for an additional 40 weeks. Following a rapid onset of action, patients treated with secukinumab 300 mg reached PASI-75 response after 12 weeks in 81.6% of all cases. In the 150 mg group, 71.6% of patients reached the PASI-75. By comparison, 4.5% of placebo-treated patients had a PASI-75 response (P<0.0001). PASI-75 response rate reached its peak of 87.8% in the secukinumab 300 mg group at week 16. In the secukinumab 300 mg group, 70% of patients had PASI-90 responses at 16 weeks, and 40% showed total clearance (PASI-100). During the maintenance phase, response rates could be sustained through the 52-weeks treatment period in 80% of the patients (PASI-75), 70% (PASI-90), and 40% (PASI-100). The incidence of serious adverse events showed no significant differences in the different groups of dosing. The most common adverse events were nasopharyngitis (20–25%), upper respiratory tract infections (11%-12%), and headache (9%).

The FIXTURE study was a head-to head-study comparing efficacy of secukinumab to etanercept within a four-arm randomization, involving 1300 patients, receiving one of two doses of secukinumab, placebo, or etanercept 50 mg twice weekly for 12 weeks, then weekly thereafter. PASI-75 response rates at week 12 were 77% and 67% in the 300 mg and 150 mg secukinumab groups, respectively, compared with 44% in the etanercept treatment group. 72.4% of patients reached the PASI-90 at week 16 with the 300 mg dose of secukinumab versus 41.5% with etanercept at 32 weeks. PASI-100 scores peaked at 36.8% after 16 weeks with secukinumab 300 mg and 13.0% at 32 weeks with etanercept. Serious adverse event rates showed no differences between secukinumab and etanercept. It has to be noted that mucocutaneous candidiasis has been reported as a complication of defects in the IL-17 pathway and was also reported in the ERASURE and FIXTURE studies. Another specific event that needs further attention in further studies is neutropenia. The exact mechanism has not been elucidated so far.

Secukinumab was associated with a rapid reduction in psoriasis symptoms, elicited significantly greater PASI-75 rates and higher rates of 0 or 1 responses on the modified investigator's global assessment than placebo at week 12, and with continued treatment was associated with sustained high response rates in a majority of patients through week 52. The FIXTURE study showed the superior efficacy of secukinumab over the TNF inhibitor etanercept over a period of 52 weeks. The investigator-assessed reduction in signs and symptoms in each study was accompanied by a reduction in patient-reported itching, pain, and scaling on the 'psoriasis symptom diary' and an improvement in the health-related quality of life on the Dermatology Life Quality Index (DLQI). In 2015, the US FDA and EMA approved secukinumab for the treatment of moderate-to-severe plaque psoriasis in adult patients who are candidates for systemic therapy or phototherapy.

General considerations in the use of biologic agents for psoriasis

When choosing between biologic agents, the clinician must take into account many factors relating to the characteristics of the patient, the disease, and the therapies under consideration. Body weight is an important covariate, explaining some of the pharmacokinetic variability observed in clinical trials. An important aspect relating to the patient is the comorbidities that may represent a relative contraindication in the case of anti-TNF-α agents, such as advanced congestive heart failure, lupus erythematosus, and other autoimmune diseases as well as the presence of demyelinating disease. In such cases, ustekinumab would be the first-line choice among biologic agents. Some evidence suggests that the risk of certain infections is somewhat lower with etanercept than with other anti-TNF-α agents, but the evidence is insufficient to allow us to extrapolate robust conclusions (or recommendations) for patients with psoriasis. Although the evidence is limited, there is more published experience with etanercept in the treatment of patients who have chronic infection with hepatitis C virus or human immunodeficiency virus (HIV) [3]; the choice of a biologic agent in such patients should be decided on a case-by-case basis and biologic therapy must be closely monitored by both the dermatologist and the physician in charge of managing the chronic infection.

Various safety aspects related to the use of TNF-α antagonists have to be recalled in everyday practice during every phase of treatment. Foremost among these is the risk of serious infection. This requires careful assessment of the indications for therapy, as well as education and monitoring of the patient. Very rare side effects of TNF-α antagonists include malignancy, especially lymphoma. Adverse effects are more common in older patients. Infections, in particular, are often more serious. If suggested by patient history or clinical or laboratory chemical tests, HIV and viral hepatitis should be excluded.

Contraception must be ensured and pregnancy ruled out in women of childbearing age. Patients should be informed that serious infections have occurred with use of the drug and that prompt medical attention is required if infection is suspected.

The costs of treating psoriasis with biologics are high, but their contribution to resolution of lesions and improved quality of life, especially in patients who are currently undertreated, might reduce the need for inpatient care and improve the outcome for patients [62]. According to Schmitt and Ford, the indirect costs of productivity lost exceed the direct costs, which may justify the use of more expensive medications [63].

Adjuvant therapies

Though there is a considerable number of active compounds for topical and systemic treatments, many patients require or demand further adjuvant treatments. These may include:
- basic topical treatments:
  - emollients;
  - urea; and
  - keratolytics, eg, salicylic acid;
- baths, climate treatment, eg, sea climate, dead sea;
- physical treatments, eg, excimer laser;
- physical exercise;
- supportive nutritional measures;
- psychological and psychosocial support; and
- patient education.

Among psoriasis experts and in most guidelines there is large agreement – supported with some literature – that these adjuvant treatments are also valuable for the overall disease management [10].

Treatment combinations and rotations

Owing to different pharmacodynamics, pharmacokinetics, and toxicities associated with various psoriasis treatments, carefully selected combination therapies may lead to greater efficacy while minimizing toxicity. A combination approach is often adopted in the treatment of PsA to improve overall treatment response, although in several cases administered in off-label use. Physicians typically reserve combinatorial approaches for treating challenging patients with psoriasis, but rigorously conducted clinical investigations on combination systemic therapies are scarce. While the approved biologic medications are highly effective in most patients with psoriasis, some patients lack response to biologic monotherapy and require combination approaches for disease control. Biologics have the potential to act synergistically in combination with other systemic treatments, and each has a distinctive safety profile compared with oral medications. To date, no evidence-based recommendations exist for the use of biologics in combination with other systemic therapeutic modalities. Selection of combination therapy depends on disease severity, previous treatment, existing comorbidities, and adverse effects. In appropriately selected patients, carefully chosen combinations may result in greater efficacy while minimizing toxicity.

The following combinations used in off-label mode have been recommended in an international consensus group (Mrowietz and coworkers) based on literature and Delphi ratings [64]:

- There is no approved indication for any combination of a biologic with conventional systemic therapies in psoriasis.
- A conventional systemic therapy can be added to biologic monotherapy with the intention to improve efficacy, optimize the risk-benefit profile, reduce the risk of immunogenicity (with MTX), and enhance long-term disease management.
- For the TNF antagonists, combination with MTX (5–15 mg/week) is safe (level of evidence 4) and increases the long-term efficacy of the treatment regimen (level of evidence 3).
- Due to the lack of evidence and the potentially increased toxicity, for example, an increased skin cancer risk, the combination of TNF

antagonists or ustekinumab with cyclosporine should be used with caution (level of evidence 5).

- The combination of etanercept 25 mg/week with acitretin showed similar efficacy as 2 x 25 mg/week etanercept monotherapy (level of evidence 2).
- The combination of acitretin with lower doses of etanercept 25 mg/week has a safety profile comparable to the monotherapy (level of evidence 3).
- The combination of adalimumab with acitretin may be considered (level of evidence 4).
- A treatment combination of MTX with ustekinumab may be used, but there are limited data on safety and efficacy (level of evidence 5).
- Data for the combination of acitretin with infliximab or ustekinumab are not currently available but an increased clinical response might also be expected (level of evidence 5).

Formerly, systemic psoriasis treatments (eg, MTX and cyclosporine) and phototherapy were applied using rotating schemes in order to minimize side effects and chronic risks. To date, there are still limitations for long-term use of cyclosporine and UV treatment. However, there is growing evidence that most treatments such as biologics can and should be applied continuously and there is no need for rotations or drug breaks [64].

Drug therapies in development

Biologics have greatly improved the treatment of moderate-to-severe plaque psoriasis, as most patients are now able to achieve an initial improvement of 75% in the PASI. However, most patients do not reach a 90% improvement and furthermore responses may be lost over time, which has shown to be the case especially for TNF-α antagonists. Several new classes of anti-psoriatic drugs are currently undergoing clinical development and potential improvements with these new therapies include attaining earlier and higher-level responses that may last over a longer period of time and targeting cytokines involved directly in psoriatic inflammation (Table 5.3).

Class/target pathway	Generic drug name/description	Current status*
Biologic agents		
TNF-α inhibition	**Adalimumab:** recombinant human IgG1 monoclonal antibody specific for human TNF	Approved for psoriasis, 2008
	Etanercept: dimeric fusion protein consisting of the extracellular ligand-binding portion of the p75 TNF receptor, linked to the Fc portion of human IgG1	Approved for psoriasis, 2004
	Infliximab: chimeric IgG1 monoclonal antibody composed of human constant and murine variable regions, specific for human TNF	Approved for psoriasis, 2006
IL-12 and IL-23 inhibition	**Ustekinumab:** human IgG1 monoclonal antibody against the p40 subunit at the IL-12 and IL-23 cytokines	Approved for psoriasis, 2008
Direct inhibition of IL-17	**Brodalumab:** fully human anti-IL-17 receptor monoclonal antibody	Phase III trials under way
	Ixekizumab: humanized anti-IL-17A monoclonal antibody	Phase III trials under way
	Secukinumab: fully human anti-IL-17A monoclonal antibody	Approved for psoriasis, 2015
IL-23 blocker	**Tildrakizumab:** humanized anti-IL-23p19 monoclonal antibody	Phase III trials under way
	Guselkumab: fully human anti-IL-23p19 monoclonal antibody	Phase III trials complete
Small molecules		
PDE-4 inhibitor	**Apremilast:** inhibitor of phosphodiesterase-4	Approved for psoriasis, 2014
JAK inhibitor	**Tofacitinib:** inhibitor of Janus kinase	Phase III trials complete

Table 5.3 Biologic agents and small molecules in psoriasis. IL, interleukin; JAK, Janus kinase; PDE-4, phosphodiesterase-4; TNF, tumor necrosis factor.

Tofacitinib

Janus-associated kinases (JAKs) are protein tyrosine kinases that include JAK1, JAK2, JAK3 and TYK2. JAKs are activating signal transducers that regulate the expression of key genes mediating keratinocyte proliferation, cell activation, and inflammation. Inflammatory and proliferative cytokines involved in the pathogenesis of psoriasis, including IL-12, IL-23, IL-17, IL-21, IL-22, IL-20, and interferons signal through the JAK/STAT pathway.

One of the most investigated selective inhibitors is tofacitinib, which suppresses JAK1 and JAK3 and, to a lesser extent, JAK2 signaling. It was developed as an immunosuppressive agent for RA, Crohn's disease, ulcerative colitis and psoriasis. In a Phase II study [65] of oral tofacitinib in patients with moderate-to-severe plaque psoriasis, a PASI-75 was achieved in 67% of patients treated with 15 mg orally twice daily at week 12. Improvement was significantly greater in tofacitinib-treated patients at all doses compared with placebo. Greater improvement was also seen in other efficacy and quality-of-life measures, including PASI-90, PGA, and DLQI for all doses. Tofacitinib was generally well tolerated although potential side effects and a still insufficiently established benefit/risk ratio in recent studies have led to a failure in achieving approval for psoriasis in Europe. The continuation of clinical studies to further elucidate the safety and benefit for patients with psoriasis is in preparation.

Brodalumab

The active compound was investigated in a Phase II trial in patients with moderate-to-severe psoriasis. Patients were randomized to one of four different doses of brodalumab or placebo for 12 weeks. The PASI-75 was achieved by 83% of the patients, 75% reached the PASI-90 and 63% showed total clearance (PASI-100) [66]. Superiority in response rates could be established by the two intermediate doses of brodalumab (140 and 210 mg, respectively) administered every 2 weeks. The vast majority of patients showed DLQI scores of 0 or 1. The adverse events reported more frequently in the brodalumab groups were nasopharyngitis (8%), upper respiratory tract infection (8%), and injection site erythema (6%) suggesting a safety profile with no significant irregularity.

However Amgen, who along with the company AstraZeneca had been developing brodalumab, has stopped developing the drug based on reports of suicidal ideation and behavior during clinical trials for the drug. AstraZeneca is still considering whether to continue with the drug development, according to a statement released by AstraZeneca. There is no suggestion yet that this is a class effect.

Ixekizumab

Ixekizumab is a humanized anti-IL-17A monoclonal antibody. Results are available from a Phase II trial [67] in which 142 patients with moderate-to-severe psoriasis were randomized to one of four subcutaneous doses of ixekizumab (10–150 mg) or placebo [68]. Patients received induction doses at baseline, 2 weeks, and 4 weeks, followed by monthly treatment at weeks 8, 12, and 16. Patients treated with the three highest doses of ixekizumab (25, 75, and 150 mg) had PASI-75 rates of 77–83% at week 12 compared to 8% in the placebo group. The week 12 PASI-90 rates ranged from between 50% and 70% for the three highest doses of ixekizumab. PASI-100 rates reached a maximum of about 40% at week 12 with the two highest doses of ixekizumab. The most frequent adverse events across all treatment groups were infection and nasopharyngitis, rates that were low and similar to placebo.

Nonserious injection site reactions were observed and occurred in 10% or fewer patients. Patients who responded early (PASI-50 at week 4) were significantly more likely to attain PASI-75 and PASI-100 responses at 8, 12, and 16 weeks than were patients who did not attain PASI-50 at 4 weeks (P<0.05 to P<0.001), which may be predictive of subsequent treatment response [69]. Participants of the 52-week open-label extension study in which all patients received 120 mg of ixekizumab every 4 weeks, showed sustained rates of PASI-75, PASI-90, and PASI-100 responses through 52 weeks [70]. Patients with chronic moderate-to-severe plaque psoriasis treated with ixekizumab had significant improvement in clinical measures during the 12-week treatment period that was rapid and sustained through to 52 weeks with continued treatment. Further studies are needed to establish the long-term safety and efficacy of ixekizumab in the treatment of psoriasis.

Tildrakizumab

Tildrakizumab is a humanized monoclonal antibody that targets the IL-23p19 subunit. In a Phase IIb clinical trial [71], 340 patients were randomized to one of four doses (5, 25, 100, and 200 mg) of tildrakizumab or placebo; 65.5% to 76.2% of patients achieved a PASI-75 for the three highest doses of tildrakizumab. In the highest dosing group,

51.2% achieved PASI-90 response at week 16. The most common adverse event was nasopharyngitis.

The rate of adverse events did not differ substantially from the placebo groups. Patients who achieved PASI-75 responses in the trial were eligible to enter an extension phase that continued to week 52. Results of the extension study showed that response to tildrakizumab remained stable out to 52 weeks. Adverse events were similar to placebo. Further results will arise from the ongoing Phase III trials.

Future outlook

With the emerging treatment options, physicians and patients may find more convenient and safer ways to achieve sustained disease control in a shorter time. Anti-TNF agents are important therapeutic options for psoriasis, but for patients in whom response is lost or does not exist, other treatment options are required.

Current data from clinical trials suggest that biologic agents targeting IL-12, IL-17, and IL-23 are safe and efficacious drugs for use in moderate-to-severe chronic plaque psoriasis. Long-term data still need to be established [72]. It is important to note that psoriasis is often associated with several comorbidities, in particular cardiovascular disease. Several risk factors for cardiovascular events have been reported in psoriasis, and some treatments for the disease appear to enhance the cardiovascular risk profile. IL-17 has been reported to be associated with atherosclerosis by favoring chronic vascular inflammation, so might contribute to the increased risk of cardiovascular disease found in patients with psoriasis [73].

The development of new treatment targets to individualize healthcare for patients with chronic inflammatory diseases is gaining rapid momentum in a heterogeneous autoinflammatory setting. In the future there will be the need of biomarkers to predict treatment outcomes and individualize care for patients with psoriasis. Systemic and biologic agents used to control psoriasis display significant variability in efficacy, and are associated with varying degrees of toxicity and cost. One of the main goals in the future will be the identification of patients less likely to respond to particular treatments in order to tailor strategies within an individualized treatment approach. To accomplish this task it will be necessary to disentangle the relationship between a genetic variability and its relationship with treatment response and the development of adverse events. Therefore, the genetic characterization of patients according to molecular mechanisms will promote the endeavor of individualized medicine. The discrepancy between ethical concerns and the need for a far-sightedness, seizing the opportunities to decode pharmacogenomics to understand the cornerstones of 'treatment-response' requires a careful and sensitive handling.

Guidelines for management of psoriasis

Evidence-based treatment guidelines can be an important tool for improving the quality of care provided to patients with psoriasis. Despite this, not all countries have their own treatment guidelines. Although the European S3 guidelines in psoriasis [74] can help to fill the gap in these countries, they cannot reflect local policies and practices. For this reason, clinicians often rate national guidelines more highly than European guidelines. Where countries do have their own guidelines, the general consensus among them can differ. For example, the absolute criteria of when to start patients with moderate-to-severe psoriasis on systemic therapies, how to measure their success and how to define non-successful therapies varies widely. In addition, both European and national guidelines provide little information on the indications for treatment switching and on how to switch, for instance, in the following circumstances:

- when a treatment has not enabled sufficient control of the disease;
- when a treatment is contraindicated due to another coexisting disease or condition;
- when a treatment is contraindicated due to co-existing medication; and
- when a patient is intolerant to a treatment.

These disparities and omissions can prove problematic for healthcare professionals (HCPs) seeking solid guidance.

In addition to guideline development, consideration needs to be given to how guidelines are practically implemented. One barrier to implementation is that many HCPs are unaware of current guidelines due to a lack of promotion and dissemination. Limited time during consultation also makes it difficult to refer to guidelines, with visits of 5–10 minutes being inadequate for the management of patients with such a complex disease; such short visiting times may reflect the lack of priority given to psoriasis as a serious medical condition.

Furthermore, limited time during a consultation also means that HCPs may struggle to give appropriate explanations about their proposed treatment approach, or demonstrate empathy towards a patient with psoriasis regarding the challenges of their disease. Both of these factors have been found to determine patient satisfaction and ultimately adherence to medication. A lack of national guidelines in some countries and lack of consensus amongst those that do exist in others is problematic. Specifically, poor and inconsistent advice on initiating and optimizing therapeutic interventions is a barrier to improving outcomes. While European guidelines can help to fill the gap in countries without national guidelines, their role should primarily be to strengthen and harmonize existing guidelines, and to provide a framework for the development of new national guidelines.

Disease management of any illness encompasses numerous aspects of health service provision including appropriate care that is timely and provided by a multidisciplinary team mostly comprising of medical, nursing, and allied health professionals. Other key elements essential for effective care include psychosocial assessment, suitable and timely referral, information provision and personalized treatment that considers the individual patient's needs and preferences. However, there are many 'supply and demand' barriers that affect access to health services in psoriasis care. The number of identified access barriers to guideline-compliant treatment and evidence-based medicine is considerable but the literature on these and on interventions to address them is disproportionally small.

Despite the availability of a number of options for the treatment of psoriasis, surveys have demonstrated that people with psoriasis do not receive the optimal care that is necessarily needed to clear their skin symptoms, treat their disease and improve their quality of life. According to a UK study [75] in a large cohort of primary care patient records, 94% were managed on topical agents, with only 0.7% having access to secondary care, even though there were signs (eg, comorbidities) indicating that their psoriasis was not optimally controlled and that they should be referred to secondary care. Although to date no direct evidence exists supporting earlier intervention with systemic therapies, psoriasis and RA share common pathogenic pathways and, as a result, parallels may be drawn. The benefit of early intervention in RA has been shown in several studies. For example, an Austrian study compared two similarly treated groups of RA patients, with the only difference being a 9-month average delay in starting therapy in the second group. The patients that received early intervention showed a significantly better response in disease activity and irreversible joint damage after 3 years of follow-up. Similarly, a British study on PsA revealed superior outcomes in patients being treated with a more stringent, goal-oriented approach compared with routine care. It is probable, therefore, that earlier therapeutic intervention in psoriasis, with early and often irreversible cumulative damage, also may help offset this kind of impairment.

References

1   Mrowietz U, Kragballe K, Reich K, et al. Definition of treatment goals for moderate-to-severe psoriasis: a European consensus. *Arch Dermatol Res*. 2011;303:1–10.
2   Reich K, Mrowietz U. Treatment goals in psoriasis. *J Dtsch Dermatol Ges*. 2007;5:566-574.
3   Strober BE, Berger E, Cather J, et al. A series of critically challenging case scenarios in moderate-to-severe psoriasis: a Delphi consensus approach. *J Am Acad Dermatol*. 2009;61:S1-S46.
4   Strober BE, Clay Cather J, Cohen D et al. A Delphi consensus approach to challenging case scenarios in moderate-to-severe psoriasis: part 1. *Dermatol Ther (Heidelb)*. 2012;2:1.
5   Strober BE, Clay Cather J, Cohen D et al. A Delphi consensus approach to challenging case scenarios in moderate-to-severe psoriasis: part 2. *Dermatol Ther (Heidelb)*. 2012;2:2.
6   Mrowietz U, de Jong EM, Kragballe K, et al. A consensus report on appropriate treatment optimization and transitioning in the management of moderate-to-severe plaque psoriasis. *J Eur Acad Dermatol Venereol*. 2014;28:438-453.
7   Augustin M, Holland B, Dartsch D, Langenbruch A, Radtke MA. Adherence in the treatment of psoriasis: a systematic review. *Dermatology*. 2011;222:363-374.
8   Neri L, Miracapillo A. Treatment adherence and real-life effectiveness of topical therapy in patients with mild or moderate psoriasis: uptake of scientific evidence in clinical practice and dermatologists' preferences for alternative treatment options. *G Ital Dermatol Venereol*. 2015;150:19-26.
9   Blome C, Simianer S, Purwins S, et al. Time needed for treatment is the major predictor of quality of life in psoriasis. *Dermatology*. 2010;221:154-159.
10   Nast A, Boehncke WH, Mrowietz U, et al. S3 - Guidelines on the treatment of psoriasis vulgaris (English version). Update. Deutsche Dermatologische Gesellschaft (DDG); Berufsverband Deutscher Dermatologen (BVDD). *J Dtsch Dermatol Ges*. 2012;10 Suppl 2:S1-S95.
11   Augustin M, Mrowietz U, Bonnekoh B, et al. Topical long-term therapy of psoriasis with vitamin D_3 analogues, corticosteroids and their two compound formulations: position paper on evidence and use in daily practice. *J Dtsch Dermatol Ges*. 2014;12:667-682.

12 Singh S, Gopal J, Mishra RN, Pandey SS. Topical 0.05% betamethasone dipropionate: efficacy in psoriasis with once a day vs. twice a day application. *Br J Dermatol*. 1995;133:497-498.

13 English JS, Bunker CB, Ruthven K, Dowd PM, Greaves MW. A double-blind comparison of the efficacy of betamethasone dipropionate cream twice daily versus once daily in the treatment of steroid responsive dermatoses. *Clin Exp Dermatol*. 1989;14:32-34

14 Reich K, Zschocke I, Bachelez H, et al. Efficacy of a fixed combination of calcipotriol/betamethasone dipropionate topical gel in adult patients with mild to moderate psoriasis: blinded interim analysis of a phase IV, multicenter, randomized, controlled, prospective study. *J Eur Acad Dermatol Venereol*. 2015;29:1156-1163.

15 Augustin M, Mrowietz U, Bonnekoh B, et al. Topical long-term therapy of psoriasis with vitamin D_3 analogues, corticosteroids and their two compound formulations: position paper on evidence and use in daily practice. *J Dtsch Dermatol Ges*. 2014;12:667-682.

16 Ma L, Yang Q, Yang H, et al. Calcipotriol plus betamethasone dipropionate gel compared with calcipotriol scalp solution in the treatment of scalp psoriasis: a randomized, controlled trial investigating efficacy and safety in a Chinese population. *Int J Dermatol*. 2015 [Epub ahead of print]; doi:10.1111/ijd.12788.

17 Schröder JM, Kosfeld U, Christophers E. Multifunctional inhibition by anthralin in nonstimulated and chemotactic factor stimulated human neutrophils. *J Invest Dermatol*. 1985;85:30-34.

18 Weinstein GD, Koo JY, Krueger GG, et al. Tazarotene cream in the treatment of psoriasis: Two multicenter, double-blind, randomized, vehicle-controlled studies of the safety and efficacy of tazarotene creams 0.05% and 0.1% applied once daily for 12 weeks. *J Am Acad Dermatol*. 2003;48:760-767.

19 Armstrong AW, Bagel J, Van Voorhees AS, Robertson AD, Yamauchi PS. Combining biologic therapies with other systemic treatments in psoriasis: evidence-based, best-practice recommendations from the Medical Board of the National Psoriasis Foundation. *JAMA Dermatol*. 2015;151:432-438.

20 Ramsay CA, Schwartz BE, Lowson D, Papp K, Bolduc A, Gilbert M. Calcipotriol cream combined with twice weekly broad-band UVB phototherapy: a safe, effective and UVB-sparing antipsoriatic combination treatment. The Canadian Calcipotriol and UVB Study Group. *Dermatology*. 2000; 200:17-24.

21 Brockow T, Schiener R, Franke A, Resch KL, Peter RU. A pragmatic randomized controlled trial on the effectiveness of highly concentrated saline spa water baths followed by UVB compared to UVB only in moderate to severe psoriasis. *J Altern Complement Med*. 2007;13: 725-732.

22 Brockow T, Schiener R, Franke A,Resch KL, Peter RU. A pragmatic randomized controlled trial on the effectiveness of low concentrated saline spa water baths followed by ultraviolet B (UVB) compared to UVB only in moderate to severe psoriasis. *J Eur Acad Dermatol Venereol*. 2007;21:1027-1037.

23 De Leeuw J, Van Lingen RG, Both H, Tank B, Nijsten T, Martino Neumann HA. A comparative study on the efficacy of treatment with 585 nm pulsed dye laser and ultraviolet B-TL01 in plaque type psoriasis. *Dermatol Surg*. 2009;35:80-91.

24 Ring J, Kowalzick L, Christophers E, et al. Calcitriol 3 microg g-1 ointment in combination with ultraviolet B phototherapy for the treatment of plaque psoriasis: results of a comparative study. *Br J Dermatol*. 2001;144:495-499.

25 Youssef RM, Mahgoub D, Mashaly HM, El-Nabarawy E, Samir N, El-Mofty M. Different narrowband. UVB dosage regimens in dark skinned psoriatics: a preliminary study. *Photodermatol Photoimmunol Photomed*. 2008;24:256-259.

26 Petrozzi JW. Topical steroids and UV radiation in psoriasis. *Arch Dermatol*.1983;119:207-210.

27 Serwin AB, Wasowicz W, Chodynicka B. Selenium supplementation, soluble tumor necrosis factor-alpha receptor type 1, and C-reactive protein during psoriasis therapy with narrowband ultraviolet B. *Nutrition*. 2006;22:860-864.

28 Coven TR, Burack LH, Gilleaudeau R, Keogh M, Ozawa M, Krueger JG. Narrowband UV-B produces superior clinical and histopathological resolution of moderate-to-severe psoriasis in patients compared with broadband UV-B. *Arch Dermatol*. 1997;133:1514-1522.

29 Snellman E, Klimenko T, Rantanen T. Randomized half-side comparison of narrowband UVB and trimethylpsoralen bath plus UVA treatments for psoriasis. *Acta Derm Venereol*. 2004;84:132-137.

30 Amornpinyokeit N, Asawanonda P. 8-Methoxypsoralen cream plus targeted narrowband ultraviolet B for psoriasis. *Photodermatol Photoimmunol Photomed*. 2006;22:285-289.

31 Gordon PM, Diffey BL, Mattews JNS, Farr PM. A randomised comparison of narrow-band TL-01 phototherapy and PUVA photochemotherapy for psoriasis. *J Am Acad Dermatol*. 1999;41:728-732.

32 Leenutaphong V, Nimkulrat P, Sudtim S. Comparison of phototherapy two times and four times a week with low doses of narrow-band ultraviolet B in Asian patients with psoriasis. *Photodermatol Photoimmunol Photomed*. 2000;16:202-206.

33 Yones SS, Palmer RA, Garibaldinos TT, Hawk JL. Randomized double-blind trial of the treatment of chronic plaque psoriasis: efficacy of psoralen-UV-A therapy vs narrowband UV-B therapy. *Arch Dermatol*. 2006;142:836-842.

34 Goldinger SM, Dummer R, Schmid P, Prinz Vavricka M, Burg G, Lauchli S. Excimer laser versus narrow-band UVB (311 nm) in the treatment of psoriasis vulgaris. *Dermatology*. 2006;213:134-139.

35 Kaur M, Oliver B, Hu J, Feldman SR. Nonlaser UVB-targeted phototherapy treatment of psoriasis. *Cutis*. 2006;78:200-203.

36 Grundmann-Kollmann M, Ludwig R, et al. Narrowband UVB and cream psoralen-UVA combination therapy for plaque-type psoriasis. *J Am Acad Dermatol*. 2004;50:734-739.

37 Parrish JA, Fitzpatrick TB, Tanenbaum L, Pathak MA. Photochemotherapy of psoriasis with oral methoxsalen and longwave ultraviolet light. *N Engl J Med*. 1974;291:1207-1211.

38 Gyulai R, Bagot M, Griffiths CE, et al. Current practice of methotrexate use for psoriasis: results of a worldwide survey among dermatologists. *J Eur Acad Dermatol Venereol*. 2015;29:224-231.

39 Menting SP, Dekker PM, Limpens J, Hooft L, Spuls PI. Methotrexate dosing regimen for plaque-type psoriasis: a systematic review of the use of test-dose, start-dose, dosing scheme, dose adjustments, maximum dose and folic acid supplementation. *Acta Derm Venereol*. 2015 [Epub ahead of print]; doi:10.2340/00015555-2081.

40 Shea B, Swinden MV, Tanjong Ghogomu E, et al. Folic acid or folinic acid for reducing side effects of methotrexate for people with rheumatoid arthritis. *Cochrane Database Syst Rev*. 2013;5:CD000951.

41 Paul C, Gallini A, Maza A, et al. Evidence-based recommendations on conventional systemic treatments in psoriasis: systematic review and expert opinion of a panel of dermatologists. *J Eur Acad Dermatol Venereol*. 2011;25:2-11.

42 Thaci D, Brautigam M, Kaufmann R, Weidinger G, Paul C, Christophers E. Body-weight-independent dosing of cyclosporine micro-emulsion and three times weekly maintenance regimen in severe psoriasis. A randomised study. *Dermatology*. 2002;205:383-388.

43 Booij MT, Van De Kerkhof PC. Acitretin revisited in the era of biologics. *J Dermatolog Treat*. 2011;22:86-89.

44 Dogra S1, Yadav S. Acitretin in psoriasis: an evolving scenario. *Int J Dermatol*. 2014;53:525-538.

45 Papp K, Reich K, Leonardi CL, et al. Apremilast, an oral phosphodiesterase 4 (PDE4) inhibitor, in patients with moderate to severe plaque psoriasis: results of a phase III, randomized, controlled trial (Efficacy and Safety Trial Evaluating the Effects of Apremilast in Psoriasis [ESTEEM] 1). *J Am Acad Dermatol*. 2015;73:37-49.

46 Reich K, Burden AD, Eaton JN, Hawkins NS. Efficacy of biologics in the treatment of moderate to severe psoriasis: a network meta-analysis of randomized controlled trials. *Br J Dermatol*. 2012;166:179-188.

47 Mease PJ, Kivitz AJ, Burch FX, Siegel EL, Cohen SB, Ory P, Salonen D, Rubenstein J, Sharp JT, Tsuji W. Eta- nercept treatment of psoriatic arthritis: safety, efficacy, and effect on disease progression. *Arthritis Rheum*. 2004;50:2264-2272

48 Moreland LW, Schiff MH, Baumgartner SW, et al. Etanercept therapy in rheumatoid arthritis. A randomized, controlled trial. *Ann Intern Med*. 1999;130:478-486.

49 Tyring S, Gordon KB, Poulin Y, et al. Long-term safety and efficacy of 50 mg of etanercept twice weekly in patients with psoriasis. *Arch Dermatol*. 2007;143:719-726.

50 Papp KA, Tyring S, Lahfa M, et al. A global phase III randomized controlled trial of etanercept in psoriasis: safety, efficacy, and effect of dose reduction. *Br J Dermatol*. 2005;152:1304-1312.

51 Leonardi CL, Powers JL, Matheson RT, et al. Etanercept as monotherapy in patients with psoriasis. *New Engl J Med*. 2003;349:2014-2022.

52 Zachariae C, Mork NJ, Reunala T, Lorentzen H, Falk E, Karvonen SL, Johannesson A, Clareus B, Skov L, Mork G, Walker S, Qvitzau S. The combination of etanercept and methotrexate increases the effectiveness of treatment in active psoriasis despite inadequate effect of methotrexate therapy. *Acta Derm Venereol*. 2008;88:495-501.

53 Menter A, Tyring SK, Gordon K, et al. Adalimumab therapy for moderate to severe psoriasis: A randomized, controlled phase III trial. *J Am Acad Dermatol*. 2008;58:106-115.

54 Saurat JH, Stingl G, Dubertret L, et al. Efficacy and safety results from the randomized controlled comparative study of adalimumab vs. methotrexate vs. placebo in patients with psoriasis (CHAMPION). *Br J Dermatol*. 2008;158:558-566.

55 Leonardi CL, Kimball AB, Papp KA, et al. Efficacy and safety of ustekinumab, a human interleukin-12/23 monoclonal antibody, in patients with psoriasis: 76-week results from a randomised, double-blind, placebo-controlled trial (PHOENIX 1). *Lancet*. 2008;371:1665-1674.

56 Papp KA, Langley RG, Lebwohl M, et al. Efficacy and safety of ustekinumab, a human interleukin-12/23 monoclonal antibody, in patients with psoriasis: 52-week results from a randomised, double-blind, placebo-controlled trial (PHOENIX 2). *Lancet*. 2008;371:1675-1684.

57 Griffiths CE, Strober BE, van de Kerkhof P, et al. Comparison of ustekinumab and etanercept for moderate-to-severe psoriasis. *N Engl J Med*. 2010;362:118-128.

58 Menter A, Feldman SR, Weinstein GD, et al. A randomized comparison of continuous vs. intermittent infliximab maintenance regimens over 1 year in the treatment of moderate-to-severe plaque psoriasis. *J Am Acad Dermatol*. 2007;56:e1-e15.

59 Reich K, Nestle FO, Papp K, et al. Infliximab induction and maintenance therapy for moderate-to-severe psoriasis: a phase III, multicentre, doubleblind trial. *Lancet*. 2005;366:1367-1374.

60 Malakouti M, Brown GE, Wang E, Koo J, Levin EC. The role of IL-17 in psoriasis. *J Dermatolog Treat*. 2015;26:41-44.

61 Langley RG, Elewski BE, Lebwohl M, et al. Secukinumab in plaque psoriasis–results of two phase 3 trials. *N Engl J Med*. 2014;371:326-338.

62 Driessen RJ, Bisschops LA, Adang EM, Evers AW, Van De Kerkhof PC, De Jong EM. The economic impact of high-need psoriasis in daily clinical practice before and after the introduction of biologics. *Br J Dermatol*. 2010;162:1324-1329.

63 Schmitt JM, Ford DE. Work limitations and productivity loss are associated with health-related quality of life but not with clinical severity in patients with psoriasis. *Dermatology*. 2006;213:102-110.

64 Mrowietz U, de Jong EM, Kragballe K, et al. A consensus report on appropriate treatment optimization and transitioning in the management of moderate-to-severe plaque psoriasis. *J Eur Acad Dermatol Venereol*. 2014;28:438-453.

65 Papp KA, Menter A, Strober B, et al. Efficacy and safety of tofacitinib, an oral Janus kinase inhibitor, in the treatment of psoriasis: a Phase 2b randomized placebo-controlled dose-ranging study. *Br J Dermatol*. 2012;167:668-677.

66 Papp KA, Leonardi C, Menter A, et al. Brodalumab, an anti-interleukin-17-receptor antibody for psoriasis. *N Engl J Med*. 2012;366:1181-1189.

67 Zhu B, Edson-Heredia E, Cameron GS, et al. Early clinical response as a predictor of subsequent response to ixekizumab treatment: results from a phase II study of patients with moderate-to-severe plaque psoriasis. *Br J Dermatol*. 2013;169:1337-1341.

68 Leonardi C, Matheson R, Zachariae C, et al. Anti-interleukin-17 monoclonal antibody ixekizumab in chronic plaque psoriasis. *N Engl J Med*. 2012;366:1190-1199.

69 Zhu B, Edson-Heredia E, Cameron GS, et al. Early clinical response as a predictor of subsequent response to ixekizumab treatment: results from a phase II study of patients with moderate-to-severe plaque psoriasis. *Br J Dermatol*. 2013;169:1337-1341.

70 Gordon KB, Leonardi CL, Lebwohl M, et al. A 52-week, open-label study of the efficacy and safety of ixekizumab, an anti-interleukin-17A monoclonal antibody, in patients with chronic plaque psoriasis. *J Am Acad Dermatol*. 2014;71:1176-1182.

71 Papp K, Thaçi D, Reich K, Riedl E, Langley RG, Krueger JG, Gottlieb AB, Nakagawa H, Bowman EP, Mehta A, Li Q, Zhou Y, Shames R. Tildrakizumab (MK-3222), an anti-interleukin-23p19 monoclonal antibody, improves psoriasis in a phase IIb randomized placebo-controlled trial. *Br J Dermatol*. 2015;173:930-939.

72 Tausend W, Downing C, Tyring S. Systematic review of interleukin-12, interleukin-17, and interleukin-23 pathway inhibitors for the treatment of moderate-to-severe chronic plaque psoriasis: ustekinumab, briakinumab, tildrakizumab, guselkumab, secukinumab, ixekizumab, and brodalumab. *J Cutan Med Surg*. 2014;18:156-169.

73 Coimbra S, Figueiredo A, Santos-Silva A. Brodalumab: an evidence-based review of its potential in the treatment of moderate-to-severe psoriasis. *Core Evid*. 2014;9:89-97.

74 Pathirana D, Ormerod AD, Saiag P, et al. European S3-guidelines on the systemic treatment of psoriasis vulgaris. *J Eur Acad Dermatol Venereol*. 2009;23:1-70. Erratum in: *J Eur Acad Dermatol Venereol*. 2010;24:117-118.

75 Gillard SE, Finlay AY. Current management of psoriasis in the United Kingdom: patterns of prescribing and resource use in primary care. *Int J Clin Pract*. 2005;59:1260-1267.

Chapter 6

Treatment of psoriatic arthritis
Musaab Elmamoun and Oliver Fitzgerald

Treatment goals

The primary goal of treating patients with psoriatic arthritis (PsA) is to maximise health-related quality of life (HRQoL), through control of symptoms, prevention of structural damage, and normalization of function and social participation [1]. Treatment goals in PsA should aim at reaching an acceptable disease state as agreed by both patient and physician [2]. In 2009, minimal disease activity (MDA) criteria, the first potential target for treatment in PsA were published. Patients reach MDA state when meeting five of the seven following criteria: tender joint count ≤1, swollen joint count ≤1, Psoriasis Area and Severity Index (PASI) ≤1 or body surface area (BSA) ≤3, patient pain visual analog score (VAS) ≤15, patient global disease activity VAS ≤20, Health Assessment Questionnaire (HAQ) ≤0.5, and tender entheseal points ≤1 [2]. MDA criteria were validated in retrospective and observational cohorts, and are increasingly used as a treatment target.

The diversity and heterogeneity of clinical manifestations in PsA (peripheral arthritis, skin and nail disease, axial disease, dactylitis, and enthesitis) add a level of complexity to therapeutic decisions because not all treatments are effective for all features. Treatment choices should be driven by the disease feature considered most severe at the time of evaluation.

© Springer International Publishing Switzerland 2016
R. Warren and A. Menter (eds.), *Handbook of Psoriasis and Psoriatic Arthritis*, DOI 10.1007/978-3-319-18227-8_6

Treatment strategy

Interventional strategy trials in PsA are lacking. Evidence is needed from Randomized Controlled Trials (RCTs) to prove benefit of early therapeutic intervention. An abstract describing the Tight Control of PsA (TICOPA) study was published in 2014. The TICOPA study showed that tight control of disease activity, in which a treat-to-target approach is used, significantly improves joint outcomes for patients newly diagnosed with PsA [3]. Two hundred and six patients with early (disease duration <24 months) disease-modifying antirheumatic drug (DMARD)-naive PsA were recruited from 2008 to 2012. One hundred and one patients were randomized to tight control with step up regimen aiming at minimal disease activity as a target, and 105 to standard care. In the intention to treat (ITT) population, the odds of achieving an American College of Rheumatology 20 (ACR20) score at 48 weeks were greater in the tight control group than in the standard control group (odds ratio [OR] 1.91, 95% confidence interval [CI] 1.03–3.55; p=0.0392). In complete case analysis, 55 (61.8%) of 89 patients in the tight control group showed ACR20 response compared with 37 (44.6%) of 83 patients receiving standard care (χ^2 5.11, p=0.02). Adverse events were reported in 179 (86.9%) of 206 patients (97% [98/101] tight control versus 77.1% [81/105] standard control) [3]. This study has shown the potential benefit of a treat-to-target approach in PsA.

Group for Research and Assessment of Psoriasis and Psoriatic Arthritis (GRAPPA) and European League Against Rheumatism (EULAR) have recently updated their guidelines and they have been submitted for publication. A proposed treatment strategy that has been developed locally, based on 2011 EULAR guidelines is outlined below [4]. Patients with mono/oligoarticular features can be treated with NSAIDs and/or intra-articular steroid injections. Patients with active polyarticular disease, particularly those with many swollen joints, structural damage in the presence of inflammation, high erythrocyte sedimentation rate (ESR)/C-reactive protein (CRP), and/or clinically relevant extra-articular manifestations, should be started on treatment with DMARDs at an early stage. In patients with active PsA and clinically relevant psoriasis, a DMARD that also improves psoriasis such as methotrexate should be preferred.

Patients with active arthritis and an inadequate response to at least one synthetic DMARD (sDMARD), should commence on treatment with a tumor necrosis factor inhibitor (TNFi).

In patients with active enthesitis and/or dactylitis and insufficient response to non-steroidal anti-inflammatory drugs (NSAIDs) or local steroid injections, TNFi may be considered. Patients who present with predominantly active axial disease and who have insufficient response to NSAIDs should be commenced on TNFi. In patients who fail to respond adequately, switching to another TNFi agent should be considered. In patients who fail TNFi therapy, ustekinumab or other novel therapies may be considered. For further details see Figure 6.1.

Treatment options for therapy in psoriatic arthritis

Available treatments for PsA include:

- NSAIDs (eg, diclofenac, naproxen, ibuprofen, celecoxib, and etricoxib);
- sDMARDs (eg, methotrexate, sulphasalazine, leflunomide and cyclosporin);
- approved biologic DMARDS (bDMARDs) that include: TNFi agents (eg, adalimumab, infliximab, etanercept, golimumab, and certolizumab pegol), the inteleukin (IL)-12/23 inhibitor ustekinumab, and the phosphodiesterase-4 (PDE4) inhibitor apremilast; and
- therapies in development such as secukinumab, brodalumab, abatacept, and ixekizumab.

Non-steroidal anti-inflammatories

NSAIDs can be used as a first-line treatment; however data regarding the usefulness of NSAIDs in PsA are limited. Cardiovascular and gastro-intestinal risks should be taken into account when prescribing NSAIDs. In one study, patients were randomized to nimesulide (100, 200, or 400 mg/day) or placebo [5]. Nimesulide doses of 200 mg or 400 mg, but not 100 mg/day, were significantly better (p=0.03) than placebo in reducing the number of tender and swollen joints, and improving physician and patient global assessment of efficacy. A parallel group study compared

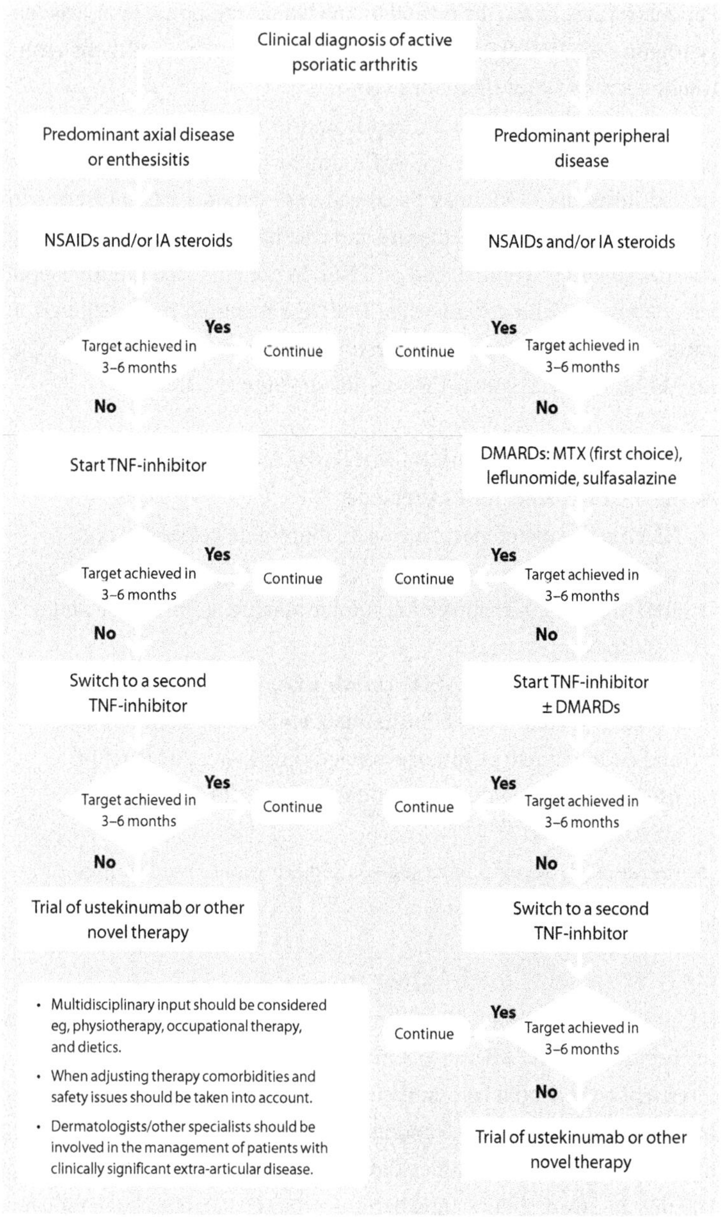

Clinical diagnosis of active
psoriatic arthritis

Predominant axial disease or enthesisitis	Predominant peripheral disease
NSAIDs and/or IA steroids	NSAIDs and/or IA steroids

Yes Target achieved in 3–6 months — Continue | Continue — **Yes** Target achieved in 3–6 months

No | **No**

| Start TNF-inhibitor | DMARDs: MTX (first choice), leflunomide, sulfasalazine |

Yes Target achieved in 3–6 months — Continue | Continue — **Yes** Target achieved in 3–6 months

No | **No**

| Switch to a second TNF-inhibitor | Start TNF-inhibitor ± DMARDs |

Yes Target achieved in 3–6 months — Continue | Continue — **Yes** Target achieved in 3–6 months

No | **No**

| Trial of ustekinumab or other novel therapy | Switch to a second TNF-inhbitor |

Continue — **Yes** Target achieved in 3–6 months

No

- Multidisciplinary input should be considered eg, physiotherapy, occupational therapy, and dietics.
- When adjusting therapy comorbidities and safety issues should be taken into account.
- Dermatologists/other specialists should be involved in the management of patients with clinically significant extra-articular disease.

Trial of ustekinumab or other novel therapy

Figure 6.1 Showing a proposed treatment strategy in patients with active psoriatic arthritis and different clinical features. IA, intra-articular; MTX, methotrexate.

celecoxib 400 mg (n=201) or celecoxib 200 mg (n=213) once daily with placebo (n=194) in treating the signs and symptoms of PsA during flare. At week 12, no statistically significant differences in ACR20 response criteria between treatment groups were observed [6]. In view of their potential toxicity, NSAIDs should be used in the lowest dose and the shortest treatment duration possible.

Corticosteroids

Intra-articular steroid injections are effective and may be a useful adjunctive therapy in localized disease, ie, mono/oligoarticular forms, enthesitis, or dactylitis. Intra-articular steroids are efficacious for mono/oligoarthritis or single joint flares, in otherwise well-controlled polyarthritis. Systemic corticosteroids are widely used in the treatment of PsA, although there is no evidence of use from clinical trials. Concerns have arisen, with some supporting case reports only, suggesting that exacerbations of psoriasis may follow corticosteroid discontinuation. The long-term use of corticosteroids can lead to major adverse events. Corticosteroids should be used in the lowest dose and the shortest duration possible, and a consideration should be given to tapering them gradually when feasible.

Synthetic disease-modifying antirheumatic drugs

Based on evidence, nearly all DMARDs may have small-to-moderate beneficial effects on peripheral joints [7]. DMARDs have no proven effects on axial disease.

Methotrexate

For many rheumatologists methotrexate remains the DMARD of first choice for patients with PsA; however evidence for its use is limited. In a randomized 6-month open-label trial in early PsA (n=35), patients were randomized to NSAIDs alone or NSAIDs plus methotrexate for 3 months; thereafter, all patients continued with NSAIDs/methotrexate [8]. Patients randomized to methotrexate had significantly ($p<0.05$) better joint count responses at 3 months compared with patients receiving NSAIDs alone, but the results were similar at 6 months when both groups were taking NSAIDs/methotrexate.

In another study [9] that included 221 patients, patients were randomized to methotrexate (7.5–15 mg weekly) or placebo. The only measure that improved significantly in the treatment group was the physician global assessment. However, this trial only allowed for a maximum dose of 15 mg/week and used Psoriatic Arthritis Response Criteria (PsARC) as a primary outcome measure, which has been shown to be associated with a high placebo response.

Leflunomide

There is good evidence for use of leflunomide from one randomized controlled trial [10]. In the trial that included 190 patients who received leflunomide or placebo for 24 weeks, 59% of patients treated with leflunomide compared with 30% of patients given placebo met the primary response criteria (PsARC). There were also significant, although small, improvements in other individual parameters, including joint scores, health assessment questionnaire results, PASI, and Dermatology Life Quality Index (DLQI) scores.

Sulfasalazine

Sulfasalazine has been shown to have a marginal effect in six randomized clinical trials. In the largest trial of 221 patients, a significantly higher percentage of patients on sulfasalazine achieved the PsARC response compared with placebo (59% of patients achieved a therapeutic response, but consistent with other studies, a high therapeutic response [42.7%] was also noted in placebo-treated patients) [11].

Cyclosporine

Cyclosporine has shown to be as effective as methotrexate; however because of its high toxicity profile, it is not widely used. In a study of 72 patients with active PsA and an incomplete response to methotrexate the addition of cyclosporine significantly improved synovitis as detected by musculoskeletal ultrasound (MSUS) and PASI score compared with placebo [12].

Hydroxychloroquine

No randomized controlled trials have been conducted to show clinical efficacy of hydroxychloroquine. There have been anecdotal reports of exacerbation of psoriasis by hydroxychloroquine; however this was not confirmed by a case-controlled study [13]. Due to concerns with exacerbation of psoriasis, hydroxychloroquine is not frequently used in PsA.

Azathioprine

There is only one controlled trial of azathioprine in PsA. A 12-month double-blind crossover study of azathioprine (3 mg/kg per day) in six patients reported moderate or marked joint improvement in all six patients and cutaneous improvement in four; however, the dose of azathioprine had to be reduced in five patients because of leukopenia. In view of known toxicity of azathioprine, appropriate monitoring is mandatory [14].

Biologic disease-modifying antirheumatic drugs

Anti-tumor necrosis factor-α

TNF-α is a potent cytokine that is critically involved in the inflammatory pathway and in joint damage in PsA. The inhibition of the effector functions of this cytokine reduces its direct action, as well as the action of other proinflammatory cytokines. A number of large, well-conducted, randomized controlled trials have accumulated evidence that TNF-α inhibitors are effective in PsA.

Etanercept

Etanercept is a soluble fusion protein composed of two P75 TNF receptor domains linked to an IgG Fc region. Patients receiving 25 mg subcutaneous twice weekly doses of etanercept showed significant improvement in ACR20 responses (59% versus 15%) at 12 weeks compared with placebo [15]. At 12 months, radiographic disease progression (modified total Sharp score) was inhibited in the etanercept group (–0.03 unit) compared with worsening of +1.00 unit in the placebo group.

Infliximab

Infliximab is a chimeric monoclonal antibody to TNF-α. Patients receiving infliximab 5 mg/kg through 24 weeks saw a significant improvement in active PsA, including dactylitis, enthesopathy, and associated psoriasis. At week 14, 58% of patients receiving infliximab and 11% of those receiving placebo achieved an ACR20 response and 77% of infliximab patients and 27% of placebo patients achieved PsARC (both p<0.001) [16].

Adalimumab

Adalimumab is a fully humanized monoclonal anti-TNF antibody. In a large randomized trial [17], 315 patients were randomly assigned to adalimumab (40 mg every other week subcutaneously) or to placebo. A significantly greater proportion of patients receiving adalimumab achieved an ACR20 response after six months of treatment (57% versus 15%). Skin disease was also better controlled by adalimumab (PASI75 achieved in 59% versus 1%). Additionally, adalimumab treatment was associated with less radiologic progression, with better QoL, and with improvement in fatigue.

Golimumab

Golimumab, a human anti-TNF-α monoclonal antibody, was effective for treating psoriasis and PsA in the multinational, double-blind, placebo-controlled GO-REVEAL trial involving 405 patients [18]. At week 14, 51% of patients receiving golimumab 50 mg and 45% of patients receiving golimumab 100 mg achieved an ACR20 response, compared with 9% of patients in placebo group (p<0.001). There was also significant skin improvement with PASI75 score achieved by 40% in the golimumab 50 mg group and 58% in the golimumab 100 mg group compared with 2.5% of the placebo group (p<0.001). In addition, improvement was noted in ACR70, HAQ, nail disease, and enthesitis. Five-year data on golimumab confirms clinical efficacy, safety, and inhibition of radiographic progression [19].

Certolizumab pegol

Certolizumab pegol is a pegylated Fc-free anti-TNF monoclonal antibody, which has also been found to be effective in treatment of PsA. In a study of 409 patients, ACR20 response was significantly greater in certolizumab pegol-treated patients receiving 200 mg every 2 weeks and 400 mg every 4 weeks when compared with placebo (58.0% and 51.9% versus 24.3% [p<0.001] at week 12) [20]. The combined certolizumab groups also exhibited significantly greater improvement in physical function at 24 weeks compared with the placebo group (change in HAQ-DI of –0.50 versus –0.19). PASI75 scores at week 48 were achieved by 66.7 and 61.8% of patients treated with 200 and 400 mg of certolizumab pegol, respectively [21]. Improvements were also observed with respect to nail disease, enthesitis, and dactylitis. Radiographic progression was also reduced at weeks 24 and 48 in patients treated with certolizumab pegol [22]. It is noteworthy, that the RAPID-PsA study is the only anti-TNF trial to include patients who were previously exposed to anti-TNF (25% of patients).

Other approved biologic disease-modifying antirheumatic drugs

Ustekinumab

Ustekinumab is a fully human IgG-1κ monoclonal antibody that binds to the common p40 subunit shared by interleukin-12 and -23. It has now been approved for psoriasis and PsA. In an RCT, 615 patients with PsA received ustekinumab 45 mg or 90 mg versus placebo at weeks 0 and 4, and every 12 weeks thereafter. At week 24, ACR20 responses were achieved by 42.4%, 49.5%, and 22.8%, respectively (p<0.0001). ACR50/70 responses were achieved by 27.9%/14.2%; 14.2%/12.2%, and 8.75%/2.4%, respectively. Further, 42.5% of all ustekinumab patients and 2.7% of placebo group (p<0.0001) achieved ≥75% improvement in the PASI (PASI75) [23], and significant improvements were observed in HAQ, dactylitis, and enthesitis, compared with placebo.

Apremilast

Apremilast is a small molecule compound that specifically inhibits PDE4, resulting in increased cyclic adenosine monophosphate (AMP) in immune cells and leading to their immunomodulation. Apremilast, the first oral biologic, has now been approved by the US Food and Drug Administration

(FDA) and European Medicines Agency (EMA) for the treatment of PsA, and is awaiting licensing in a number of countries [24]. At week 16, more patients receiving apremilast 20 mg twice daily (31%) and 30 mg twice daily (40%) achieved ACR20 versus placebo (19%) (p<0.001). Apremilast demonstrated an acceptable safety profile and was generally well tolerated [25].

Therapies in development

Secukinumab

There is accumulating evidence that interleukin-17 is central to the pathogenesis of PsA. The blockade of IL-17A has been proposed as a therapeutic target in the treatment of PsA. Secukinumab is a fully human, high-affinity, anti-IL-17A monoclonal antibody that binds to and neutralizes IL-17A. Three hundred and ninety seven patients were randomly assigned to receive secukinumab 300 mg (n=100), 150 mg (n=100), 75 mg (n=99), or placebo (n=98). A significantly higher proportion of patients achieved an ACR20 at week 24 with secukinumab 300 mg (54 [54%] patients; odds ratio versus placebo 6.81, 95% CI 3.42–13.56; p<0.0001), 150 mg (51 [51%] patients; 6.52, 3.25–13.08; p<0.0001), and 75 mg (29 [29%] patients; 2.32, 1.14–4.73; p=0.0399) versus placebo (15 [15%] patients) [26]. Secukinumab 300 mg and 150 mg improved the signs and symptoms of PsA, suggesting that secukinumab is a potential future treatment option for patients with PsA.

Brodalumab

Inhibition of IL-17 signaling by brodalumab – a human monoclonal antibody against IL-17 receptor A – also induced significant clinical responses in patients with psoriasis. In a recent study [27] in patients with PsA, ACR20 response at week 12 was achieved in 37% and 39% in patients receiving 2 doses of brodalumab versus 18% receiving placebo. These findings show that IL-17 receptor A is a potential target for the treatment of PsA, with the inhibition of downstream pathways associated with improvements in arthritis, psoriasis, and physical function. Due to concerns with serious adverse events, however, this drug development program is currently either suspended (Amgen) or under review (AstraZeneca).

Abatacept

Abatacept is a soluble, fully human fusion protein consisting of the extracellular domain of CTLA-4 (cytotoxic T-lymphocyte antigen-4) linked to a modified Fc portion of human IgG1. Abatacept is selectively designed to interfere with T-cell co-stimulation.

In an RCT evaluating three dosing regimens of intravenous abatacept in 170 patients with PsA, 10 mg/kg abatacept administered concomitantly with DMARD was associated with improvement in both joint and skin symptoms. At 6 months, mean (SD) changes from baseline in magnetic resonance imaging (MRI) scores for erosion, osteitis, and synovitis were: -0.6 ± 4.2, -1.1 ± 2.6, and -1.4 ± 3.0, respectively, in the 10 mg/kg arm versus 1.5 ± 7.4, 0.4 ± 3.3, and 0.8 ± 4.3, respectively, in the placebo arm [28].

Ixekizumab

Ixekizumab is a monoclonal antibody with high affinity and specificity that binds to and neutralizes the pro-inflammatory cytokine IL-17A. Ixekizumab has been shown to improve psoriasis [29]. A Phase III randomized, active- and placebo-controlled study (SPIRIT-P1) examining the effect of ixekizumab compared with placebo in patients with active PsA who are bDMARD-naive is ongoing [30].

Surgery

There is a paucity of data concerning the role of surgery in patients with PsA. In one retrospective study (n=440), 7% of patients with PsA had undergone musculoskeletal surgery after an average of 13.9 years after the diagnosis of joint disease [31]. Factors predictive of subsequent surgery included the presence of radiographic damage and the number of actively inflamed joints. The probability for surgery increased with disease duration. Joint replacements have been performed when PsA leads to joint damage that leads to functional impairment [32]. A review of the types of procedures performed in a cohort of patients with PsA documented the following [33]:

• patients with oligoarticular disease usually underwent hip or knee surgery;

- patients with distal joint disease usually had hand surgery; and
- patients with polyarticular disease underwent a variety of procedures.

There was no clear evidence to suggest that patients with PsA in this study had any increased risk of infection, only one infection is reported in 71 procedures. Hicken and colleagues [34] reported that wrists and proximal interphalangeal were the most severely affected although the distal interphalangeal involvement was more common in PsA compared with rheumatoid arthritis (RA). Fusion of the distal and proximal interphalangeal joints was frequently performed. The most common surgical procedure for psoriatic foot was forefoot arthroplasty.

Quality of life in psoriatic arthritis

PsA increases the disease burden associated with psoriasis by further diminishing QoL and causing progressive joint damage. Several studies [35–38] have shown that clinical features of PsA including comorbid condition and disease activity, lead to a reduced physical and psychosocial HRQoL as compared with the general population. Patients with PsA have significantly worse physical QoL, including physical disability and pain, compared with psoriasis patients, as reflected by the Physical Component Summary (PCS) score of Short Form (SF) questionnaire and HAQ-disability index. Rosen et al [37] have shown that patients with PsA have more functional disability and reduced quality of life, measured by all questionnaires except DLQI, compared with patients with psoriasis only.

There is evidence from clinical trials to suggest that treatment of PsA improves QoL. Saad and colleagues have shown that, in addition to controlling disease activity, TNF inhibitors can significantly improve physical disability and quality of life. Greatest improvements were seen in the SF-36 PCS and the HAQ, with smaller improvements observed in the SF-36 Mental Component Summary (MCS) [39].

Finally, treatment options for PsA continue to expand and new biological therapies, both available and in development, mean that PsA patients are reaching levels of disease control previously not thought possible. However, biological therapies are expensive and place a huge cost burden on health systems. It is also noteworthy that some patients do not respond to biologics and some may lose efficacy with time or develop intolerable side effects.

Finally, PsA is associated with a number of co-morbidities that need to be addressed when managing patients with PsA. The risk of having myocardial infarction, diabetes, hypertension, and dyslipidemia was found to be increased in PsA. A number of studies have also highlighted the association of obesity and metabolic syndrome in PsA [40–43]. Cardiovascular disease and comorbidities should be addressed when treating PsA patients. However, we must carefully discriminate between comorbidities associated with PsA versus those that are associated with and/or modified by co-existing cardiovascular risks and arthritis treatment. EULAR has published recommendations for cardiovascular risk management in patients with inflammatory arthritis based on systematic literature review. The reader is referred to this publication for a detailed review of the evidence [44]. Recommendations for treatment of common comorbidities in PsA have been developed by GRAPPA, although these recommendations are unpublished as of yet.

References

1   Smolen JS, Braun J, Dougados M, et al. Treating spondyloarthritis, including ankylosing spondylitis and psoriatic arthritis, to target: recommendations of an international task force. *Ann Rheum Dis*. 2014;73:6-16.

2   Coates LC, Cook R, Lee KA, et al. Frequency, predictors, and prognosis of sustained minimal disease activity in an observational psoriatic arthritis cohort. *Arthritis Care Res (Hoboken)*. 2010;62:970.

3   Coates LC, Moverley AR, McParland L, et al. Effect of tight control of inflammation in early psoriatic arthritis (TICOPA): a UK multicentre, open-label, randomised controlled trial. *Lancet*. 2015; [Epub ahead of print] doi: 10.1016/S0140-6736(15)00347-5.

4   Elmamoun M, Ni Mhuircheartaigh O, Kane D, et al. National recommendations for the treatment of psoriatic arthritis. *Ir J Med Sci*. 2014;184(Suppl 6):Abstract 43 (14A144).

5   Sarzi-Puttini P, Santandrea S, Boccassini L, et al. The role of NSAIDs in psoriatic arthritis: evidence from a controlled study with nimesulide. *Clin Exp Rheumatol*. 2001;19:S17-S20.

6   Kivitz AJ, Espinoza LR, Sherrer YR, Liu-Dumaw M, West CR. A comparison of the efficacy and safety of celecoxib 200 mg and celecoxib 400 mg once daily in treating the signs and symptoms of psoriatic arthritis. *Semin Arthritis Rheum*. 2007;37:164-173.

7   Soriano ER, McHugh NJ. Therapies for peripheral joint disease in psoriatic arthritis: a systematic review. *J Rheumatol*. 2006;33:1422–1430.

8   Scarpa R, Peluso R, Atteno M, et al. The effectiveness of a traditional therapeutical approach in early psoriatic arthritis: Results of a pilot randomised 6-month trial with methotrexate. *Clin Rheumatol*. 2008;27:823-826.

9 Kingsley GH, Kowalczyk A, Taylor H, et al. A randomized placebo-controlled trial of methotrexate in psoriatic arthritis. *Rheumatology (Oxford)*. 2012; 51:1368-1377.

10 Kaltwasser JP, Nash P, Gladman D, et al. Efficacy and safety of leflunomide in the treatment of psoriatic arthritis and psoriasis: a multinational, double-blind, randomized, placebo-controlled clinical trial. *Arthritis Rheum*. 2004;50:1939–1950.

11 Clegg DO, Reda DJ, Mejias E, et al. Comparison of sulfasalazine and placebo in the treatment of psoriatic arthritis. A Department of Veterans Affairs Cooperative Study. *Arthritis Rheum*. 1996;39:2013–2020.

12 Fraser AD, van Kuijk AW, Westhovens R, et al. A randomised, double blind, placebo controlled, multicentre trial of combination therapy with methotrexate plus ciclosporin in patients with active psoriatic arthritis. *Ann Rheum Dis*. 2005;64:859-864.

13 Gladman DD, Blake R, Brubacher B, Farewell VT. Chloroquine therapy in psoriatic arthritis. *J Rheumatol*. 1992;19:1724-1726.

14 Levy J, Paulus HE, Barnett EV, et al. A double-blind controlled evaluation of azathioprine treatment in rheumatoid arthritis and psoriatic arthritis. *Arthritis Rheum*.1972;15:116-117.

15 Mease PJ, Kivitz AJ, Burch FX, et al. Etanercept treatment of psoriatic arthritis: safety, efficacy, and effect on disease progression. *Arthritis Rheum*. 2004;50:2264–2272.

16 Antoni C, Krueger GG, de Vlam K, et al. Infliximab improves signs and symptoms of psoriatic arthritis: results of the IMPACT 2 trial. *Ann Rheum Dis*. 2005;64:1150-1157.

17 Mease PJ, Gladman DD, Ritchlin CT, et al. Adalimumab for the treatment of patients with moderately to severely active psoriatic arthritis: results of a double-blind, randomized, placebo controlled trial. *Arthritis Rheum*. 2005;52:3279-3289.

18 Kavanaugh A, McIness I, Mease P, et al. Golimumab, a new human tumor necrosis factor α antibody, administered every 4 weeks as a subcutaneous injection in psoriatic arthritis: Twenty-four-week efficacy and safety results of a randomized, placebo-controlled study. *Arthritis Rheum*. 2009;60:976-986.

19 Kavanaugh A, McInnes IB, Mease P, et al. Clinical efficacy, radiographic and safety findings through 5 years of subcutaneous golimumab treatment in patients with active psoriatic arthritis: results from a long-term extension of a randomised, placebo-controlled trial (the GO-REVEAL study). *Ann Rheum Dis*. 2014;73:1689-1694.

20 Mease PJ, Fleischmann R, Deodhar AA, et al. Effect of certolizumab pegol on signs and symptoms in patients with psoriatic arthritis: 24-week results of a Phase 3 double-blind randomized placebo-controlled study (RAPID-PsA). *Ann Rheum Dis*. 2014;73:48-55.

21 Mease PJ, Fleischmann RM, Wollenhaupt J, et al. Effect of certolizumab pegol over 48 weeks 0n signs and symptoms in patients with psoriatic arthritis with and without prior tumor necrosis factor inhibitor exposure. Abstract # 312. *Arthritis Rheum*. 2013;S132.

22 Van der Heijde D, Fleischmann R, Wollenhaupt J, et al. Effect of different imputation approaches on the evaluation of radiographic progression in patients with psoriatic arthritis: result of the RAPID-PsA 24-weekphase III double-blind randomised placebo-controlled study of certolizumab pegol. *Ann Rheum Dis*. 2014;73:233-237.

23 McInnes IB, Kavanaugh A, Gottlieb AB, et al. Efficacy and safety of ustekinumab in patients with active psoriatic arthritis: 1 year results of the phase 3, multicentre, double-blind, placebo-controlled PSUMMIT 1 trial. *Lancet*. 2013;382:780-789.

24 FitzGerald O. Spondyloarthropathies: apremilast: welcome advance in treatment of psoriatic arthritis. *Nat Rev Rheumatol*. 2014;10:385-386.

25 Kavanaugh A, Mease PJ, Gomez-Reino JJ, et al. Treatment of psoriatic arthritis in a phase 3 randomized, placebo-controlled trial with apremilast, an oral phosphodiesterase 4 inhibitor. *Ann Rheum Dis*. 2014;73:1020-1026.

26 McInnes IB, Mease PJ, Kirkham B, et al. Secukinumab, a human anti-interleukin-17A monoclonal antibody, in patients with psoriatic arthritis (FUTURE 2): a randomised, double-blind, placebo-controlled, phase 3 trial. *Lancet*. 2015 [Epub ahead of print]; doi:10.1016/S0140-6736(15)61134-5.

27 Mease PJ, Genovese MC, Greenwald MW, et al. Brodalumab, an anti-IL17RA monoclonal antibody, in psoriatic arthritis. *N Engl J Med*. 2014;370:2295-2306.

28 Mease P, Genovese MC, Gladstein G, et al. Abatacept in the treatment of patients with psoriatic arthritis: Results of a six-month, multicenter, randomized, double-blind, placebo-controlled, phase II trial. *Arthritis Rheum*. 2011;63:939-948.

29 Leonardi C, Matheson R, Zachariae C, et al. Anti-interleukin-17 monoclonal antibody ixekizumab in chronic psoriasis. *N Engl J Med*. 2012;366:1190-1199.

30 Eli Lilly and Company. A Study of Ixekizumab in Participants With Active Psoriatic Arthritis (SPIRIT-P1). https://clinicaltrials.gov/ct2/show/NCT01695239. Accessed October 15, 2015.

31 Zangger P, Gladman DD, Bogoch ER. Musculoskeletal surgery in psoriatic arthritis. *J Rheumatol*. 1998;25:725-729.

32 Lambert JR, Wright V. Surgery in patients with psoriasis and arthritis. *Rheumatol Rehabil*. 1979;18:35-37.

33 Zangger P, Esufali ZH, Gladman DD, et al. Type and outcome of reconstructive surgery for different patterns of psoriatic arthritis. *J Rheumatol*. 2000;27:967-974.

34 Hicken GJ, Kitaoka HB, Valente RM. Foot and ankle surgery in patients with psoriasis. *Clin Orthop Relat Res*. 1994;300:201-206.

35 Husted JA, Tom BD, Farewell VT, Schentag CT, Gladman DD. A longitudinal study of the effect of disease activity and clinical damage on physical function over the course of psoriatic arthritis: does the effect change over time? *Arthritis Rheum*. 2007;56:840-849.

36 Dalal DS, Lin YC, Brennan DM, Borkar N, Korman N, Husni ME. Quantifying harmful effects of psoriatic disease on quality of life: cardio-metabolic outcomes in psoriatic arthritis study (COMPASS). *Semin Arthritis Rheum*. 2015;44:641-645.

37 Rosen CF, Mussani F, Chandran V, Eder L, Thavaneswaren A, Gladman DD. Patients with psoriatic arthritis have worse quality of life than those with psoriasis alone. *Rheumatology (Oxford)*. 2012;51:571-576.

38 Lee S, Mendelsohn A, Sarnes E. The burden of psoriatic arthritis: a literature review from a global health systems perspective. *PT*. 2010;35:680-689.

39 Saad AA, Ashcroft DM, Watson KD, et al. Improvement in quality of life and functional status in patients with psoriatic arthritis receiving anti-tumor necrosis factor therapies. *Arthritis Care Res (Hoboken)*. 2010;62:345-353.

40 Eder L, Jayakar J, Shanmugarajah S, et al. The burden of carotid artery plaques is higher in patients with psoriatic arthritis compared with those with psoriasis alone. *Ann Rheum Dis*. 2013;72:715-720.

41 Mok C, Ko G, Ho L, et al. Prevalence of atherosclerotic risk factors and the metabolic syndrome in patients with chronic inflammatory arthritis. *Arthritis Care Res*. 2011;62:19-202.

42 Haroon M, Gallagher P, Heffernan E, et al. High prevalence of metabolic syndrome and of insulin resistance in psoriatic arthritis is associated with the severity of underlying disease. *J Rheumatol*. 2014;41:1357-1365.

43 Jamnitski A, Symmons D, Peters MJ, et al. Cardiovascular comorbidities in patients with psoriatic arthritis: a systematic review. *Ann Rheum Dis*. 2013;72:211-216.

44 Peters MJ, Symmons DP, McCarey D, et al. EULAR evidence-based recommendations for cardiovascular risk management in patients with rheumatoid arthritis and other forms of inflammatory arthritis. *Ann Rheum Dis*. 2010;69:325-331.

Chapter 7

Quality of life in psoriasis
Matthias Augustin and Marc Alexander Radtke

Background

Psoriasis can affect health-related quality of life (HRQoL) to an extent similar to the effects of other severe chronic diseases such as depression, myocardial infarction, cancer, or hypertension [1]. The visible nature of psoriasis can be particularly disabling [2], with evidence of stigma, lowered self-image, depression, anxiety, and suicidal ideation [3] even in mild psoriasis [1]. Psychological impairment has been observed in social settings and in the workplace [4,5]. Research has shown that patients with psoriasis report physical discomfort, impaired emotional functioning, a negative body and self-image, and limitations in their daily activities, social contacts, skin-exposing activities, and work [6,7]. It has become evident that psoriasis may increase the risk of other chronic diseases, as associations with cardiovascular disease, Type 2 diabetes, obesity, and metabolic syndrome are established. Growing literature on comorbidity risks in psoriasis [8] and increased understanding of the immunopathology of psoriatic inflammation has, moreover, redefined psoriasis as chronic systemic inflammation, especially in patients with a moderate-to-severe course of disease [9,10]. Another medically and socio-economically important fact is that psoriasis patients live with their disease for periods of up to several decades. Understanding the key risk factors for patient illness perception may help physicians to identify patients who are more vulnerable to the cumulative impact of psoriasis,

© Springer International Publishing Switzerland 2016
R. Warren and A. Menter (eds.), *Handbook of Psoriasis
and Psoriatic Arthritis*, DOI 10.1007/978-3-319-18227-8_7

thereby resulting in more appropriate treatment decisions early in the course of the disease [6,11].

Many studies have shown that there is a discrepancy between the effective psoriasis treatments available and the current care situation [12–14]. Psoriatic care is far from being satisfactory: many treatments show low efficacy, have marked side effects, or are time consuming [15] leading to a high burden of disease. Surveys in a number of countries have revealed a substantial under-treatment of patients with moderate-to-severe psoriasis, leaving a considerable proportion without adequate disease control. In addition, a high number of patients were not satisfied with their treatment, including the time they needed to allocate for skin therapy and the number of visits to physicians [1]. Thus, modern psoriasis therapies should not only show good efficacy, but also have an impact on patient-reported outcomes (PRO), ie, increase HRQoL and provide benefit for the patients. Determination of PRO in clinical trials has become more and more important during the last years, as regulatory bodies in many countries consider patient-relevant criteria when deciding about reimbursement of new therapies.

Health-related quality of life: a multidimensional concept

HRQoL is a multidimensional construct that reflects the personal situation of an individual in life related to health. Important domains of HRQoL are the physical, emotional, social, functional, and spiritual well-being of a person. HRQoL in psoriasis is thus influenced by social stigmatization, high stress levels, physical limitations, depression, employment problems, and other psychosocial conditions including social anxiety and negative coping abilities, and a cumulative life course impairment. QoL in psoriasis is not strongly proportional to, or indeed predicted by, clinical disease severity such as the body surface area (BSA) or plaque severity measured by Psoriasis Area and Severity Index (PASI) [6,16,17]. However, satisfaction with treatment and the achievement of treatment goals seem to be predictors of QoL. Accordingly, these components could be potential targets of early intervention to avoid long-term QoL losses and thus avoid cumulative life course impairment (CLCI) [18]. Although growing evidence on the psychological distress is becoming convincing [17], physicians often do not address individual impact in psoriasis patients in routine care [19–21].

Measurement of quality of life

HRQoL is commonly measured by self-assessment questionnaires that evaluate either the generic [22–24], condition/dermatology-specific [25,26], or disease-specific [27,28] QoL. Numerous publications have shown that both generic as well as disease-specific HRQoL are significantly impaired in patients suffering from psoriasis [13,29]. To employ an independent measure of patient-reported psoriasis severity, many national as well as European guidelines and consensus statements include an assessment of HRQoL [26,30,31].

Although several HRQoL instruments are available (eg, Dermatology Life Quality Index [DLQI], Skindex-29, and Short Form-36 [SF-36]) and country-specific differences in the preferred validated instrument exist, until now, the DLQI in most studies has been most frequently used as an indicator of HRQoL because of its widespread use and simplicity [31–33]. Nevertheless, this instrument shows a variety of shortcomings that need to be known before use and interpretation.

Factors influencing the quality of life of a patient

There is evidence that HRQoL impairment may depend not only on disease severity but also be negatively influenced by younger age, initial lesions on nails, skin lesions on visible areas such as head/neck, and involvement of the genitals/groin as well as hand and foot regions [7,34–37].

Stigmatization

Psoriasis is a stigmatizing condition. Stigma is a perceived severe social disapproval based on a distinguishing condition that may arise from uninformed public attitudes as well as feelings arising from discriminations or perceived feelings from the therapy itself. Ginsburg and Link [38] identified six dimensions of stigmatization, consisting of 'anticipation of rejection', 'feeling of being flawed', 'sensitivity to others' attitudes', 'guilt and shame', 'secretiveness' and 'positive attitudes'. They do have major implications for healthcare [39]. Especially in skin diseases, visible lesions can cause feelings of stigmatization that often lead to psychological stress and social withdrawal. Even patients with relatively mild symptoms may experience high stigmatization with significantly high correlations with HQoL. Women do report stigmatization experiences more frequently than men, although in some dimensions there can be found higher values of women concerning 'specifically anticipated rejection', 'guilt and shame', and 'depression'.

Social functioning and influence on relationships

Social functioning is the ability of the individual to interact in the normal or usual way in society and can be used as a measure of quality of care [40]. It includes issues such as social contacts and activities, partnership, sexual behavior, skin-exposing social activities, sports, work, and career. Social contacts and activities in particular can include contact with family, friends, and neighbors, activities in groups, physical recreation and activities, going out socially, and going to public places were an individual has been found to be adversely affected. Personal relationships in particular can include the individual's relationship with family members, relatives and friends as well as the establishment of new friendships and social contacts appearing to be impaired. Gaikwad et al [41] showed that psoriasis affected the social functioning of 48% patients, led to decreased work efficiency in 51.1%, and to subjective distress at work in 62.8% of patients. Stress in the home environment and interpersonal relationships was reported by 69.8%. Social and occupational functioning worsened with increasing severity of psoriasis after a 1-year duration of illness. In other studies, patients with psoriasis stated feelings of embarrassment, shame, and anger influencing them in their overall behavior and leading to an avoidance of public places, reducing social life, and the possibility of social interaction [42]. Relationships with family members can be particularly affected to a high extent. In addition, 70% reported life impairment due to treatment consequences and care duties (eg, increase of stress in the relationship), 57% reported life impairment due to psychological impact (eg, worry and concern about the patient's condition), 55% reported life impairment due to social disruption (eg, reduced and limited attendance of social functions), 44% reported life impairment due to sport and leisure limitations (eg, limitations of holiday plans, sporting and leisure activities, and nights out), 37% reported life impairment due to limitations on daily activities (eg, shopping and sleep disturbances), and 37 % reported life impairment on the personal relationship with the patient (eg, increase of stress in the relationship) [43]. There is evidence that patients with lower levels of quality of life had partners with higher levels of depressive and anxious symptoms. The results highlight the importance of incorporating family variables in psychological interventions in psoriasis care, particularly family coping, and dyadic adjustment as well as the need for psychological intervention to focus both on patients and partners [44].

Localization of psoriasis

Timotijevic et al [45] demonstrated that patients with localized psoriasis of the soles had impaired QoL measured by all three instruments (EQ visual analog scale [EQ VAS], DLQI, and psoriasis disability index [PDI]), while no association between QoL measures and localization of psoriasis on the face and palms were identified.

In some studies, a higher PASI score was associated with a more impaired QoL. However, connection between PASI and DLQI in most cases was weak. Localization of psoriasis on the soles particularly affected mobility, symptoms (eg, pain, discomfort, itching), and feelings. Psoriatic arthritis (PsA) and bleeding were both associated with impaired mobility and usual daily activities, arthritis additionally with impairment in work, school, and leisure activities; while bleeding had a negative impact on symptoms, feelings, and treatment [45]. Other studies have shown that patients with affected areas involving the face and the neck were more likely to be affected socially and psychologically than patients with lesions not visible at first sight [46]. Picardi et al found that in particular women who had skin lesions on visible parts of the body were more vulnerable for psychiatric morbidity [44].

Early onset of psoriasis

Lower levels of distress have been reported with longer disease duration, which may indicate psychological acceptance or reflect long-term adaptation and avoidance of activities that trigger distress. Nevertheless, early onset of disease may affect patients in a more vulnerable phase, especially when occurring in children or young adolescents [18]. Especially in Type 1 psoriasis, which represents nearly 75% of all cases, onset of disease may occur at early childhood and adolescence. According to the younger age there may be less intrapersonal adaptive mechanisms, which may serve to protect from personality damage. Children who find themselves in a continuous process of development concerning their individual personality suffer from both the negative reactions of peers and from a possible influence of disease onset with pivotal life events, such as schooling, choice of profession, first social contacts, and partnerships [47].

Negative impact on work and profession

Psoriasis may reduce a person's ability to work and has a negative impact on their income levels [48]; the effects of psoriasis in the workplace have been shown in several studies. Moderate-to-severe psoriasis may not only have an influence on productivity but also on the ability to find employment. The choice of employment or career, and therefore income, is affected by psoriasis [49–51] and there seems to be an inverse relationship between psoriasis severity, employment, and income [52–54]. Augustin et al showed, that 39.3% of patients were unemployed due to the severity of their disease and a further 6.8% were unable to work due to plaque-type psoriasis [29]. Another investigation revealed absenteeism from work due to psoriasis in 60% of the patients with an average of 26 working days per year [55]. Feldman et al [56] and Pearce et al [53] established correlations between disease severity and impact on work. Ayala et al [48] recently evaluated the impact of psoriasis on education prospects and work limitations in 787 patients and found that 55% had limited expectations of career progression, 42% reported that psoriasis reduced the prospects of improvement in employment status, and 35% stated to have reduced earning potential. Another 60% of patients reported psoriasis localized to their hands and feet causing work limitations and in 25% of the cases causing them to quit their jobs. In view of the physical and mental discomfort that psoriasis can cause, people with the condition need to think carefully about their choice of career. Professions that involve social interactions to a high extent can also be potentially stressful, which represents a significant socioeconomic problem.

Time for treatment

In a study conducted by Blome et al [15], the highest predictive parameter for QoL reductions was the time needed for psoriasis treatment every day. The authors discussed several possible explanations for this relationship. First, treatment efforts in daily living could directly impair the HRQoL of patients with psoriasis: daily treatment leaves less time for other activities, patients might feel more inflexible as they have to stay on their treatment schedule, or treatment might directly exclude them from participation in certain activities. Furthermore, more treatment time could derive from more burdensome treatments; for example, to many patients topical treatment is not only more time-consuming than systemic treatment but it is also more uncomfortable. Moreover, treating the lesions reminds them of their psoriasis and is perceived itself as a stigmatizing moment. Patients might seek to forget the affliction and lead a normal life as far as possible; however, treatment could force them to focus on their condition.

Illness perception

Patients with greater disease severity have stronger health beliefs about the chronicity of psoriasis, its negative consequences, and its emotional impact. Although studies have shown in contrast that the overall PASI was not associated with patients' belief about the cause, cure/control, consequences, chronicity, or symptoms perceived [3]. Wahl et al [6] demonstrated that patients who had more 'knowledge' and higher education had less perceived consequences of psoriasis and a better personal understanding of the disease. Knowledge refers to 'psoriasis knowledge'; in the cited study it has been measured by the The Psoriasis Knowledge Questionnaire (PKQ), which was developed in a Norwegian dermatology context. The PKQ contains 49 questions about psoriasis (its etiology, development, and treatments) that patients are required to answer. The questionnaire constitutes an additive index that contains 49 items related to issues such as disease characteristics, causes, and effects on disease development, treatment, and the characteristics of prevalence. There are three response options for each statement: "valid", "uncertain," and "invalid". The total score is calculated based on the number of correct responses, with a possible range of 0–49. As the PKQ is an additive index, assessments of dimensionality (factor analysis) are not considered appropriate psychometric approaches. Higher scores indicate higher levels of knowledge. Those who felt competent and in control of their life may have more effective coping strategies when facing challenges posed by a chronic illness. Kotsis et al [57] showed in patients with joint involvement that the prevalence of moderate-to-severe levels of depressive symptoms (PHQ-9 score $\geq$10) was 21.7% in PsA patients, 25.1% in rheumatoid arthritis (RA) patients, and 36.7% in those PsA patients with polyarthritis. After adjustment for severity of disease and pain, anxiety and concern about bodily symptoms attributed to the illness were independent correlates of physical HRQoL in PsA.

Comorbidities

It is well known from countless studies that patients with psoriasis carry an increased risk of developing comorbidities related to the metabolic syndrome which includes arterial hypertension, adiposity and abnormalities in lipid and glucose metabolism [8]. This association is believed to account, at least partially, for the higher rate of cardiovascular complications observed among patients with psoriasis and to contribute to the decreased life expectancy observed in patients with severe disease. Moreover, depression is a major comorbidity of psoriasis (10–62%), which is accompanied by a distinct deterioration of the care indicators of psoriasis (number of days ill or unable to work and office visits). Suicidal thoughts are reported with significantly greater frequency than in other dermatological diseases. The prevalence of depression correlates negatively with treatment adherence [58,59]. Apart from the fact that they may trigger or aggravate psoriasis, comorbid diseases may, by their own nature, be aggravating factors for patient burden and cumulation of life impairment. In conclusion, there are already several reasons to recommend screening psoriasis patients for comorbidities. One more reason is the impact of comorbidities on HRQoL. Evidence-based recommendations for screening have been published [60] and screening algorithm tools are in the process of development [61].

Physical implications

Evidence supports that psoriasis is not only associated with psychological distress but also displays a physical impact. Skin discomfort was reported by up to 37% of psoriasis patients and skin pain by up to 42% [62–64]. Studies also showed that psoriasis-related skin symptoms are associated with sleep disturbance [65–67] and psychological distress [3,68,69], and result in an impaired HRQoL [68,70]. Ljosaa et al [71] investigated the association between skin pain or skin discomfort and HRQoL, and explored whether sleep disturbance and psychological distress were mediators of these associations. A total of 139 psoriasis patients from a university hospital setting participated in this exploratory, cross-sectional study. Data were obtained through interviews and questionnaires (DLQI, General Sleep Disturbance Scale, and Illness Perception Questionnaire) and analyzed using a series of multiple regression analyses. HRQoL was the dependent variable. Independent variables and assumed mediators were entered into the model in a predefined order. Skin pain, skin discomfort, sleep disturbance, and psychological distress were significantly associated with HRQoL (all $p<0.05$). Sleep disturbance was a partial mediator for the association between skin pain and HRQoL. In this study, skin pain and skin discomfort were significantly related to HRQoL when controlling for demographic and clinical characteristics. In addition, sleep disturbance mediated the association between skin pain and HRQoL. The results underlined the importance of the association between physiological and psychological factors, and the necessity to incorporate these findings in concepts of health care provision [71].

Goal attainment scaling and patient benefit index

There is strong evidence that HRQoL in psoriasis treatment – as with other diseases – is associated with the patient's perception of attaining the goals of the therapy applied [72]. For this, a systematic assessment methodology for measuring patient goals and needs in treatment and the degree of goal achievements was developed [18,26,73]. The overall benefit from treatment – indexed as 'Patient benefit index' is highly predictive for QoL, patient satisfaction, and patient reported benefits from treatment [73]. It is also more predictive for the overall patient benefit than clinical outcomes such as delta PASI or delta BSA [74].

Concept of cumulative life course impairment

The concept of CLCI is the result of a life-long interaction between the main influencing factors of HRQoL in patients with psoriasis, such as stigmatization, physical, and psychological comorbidity as well as coping strategies and external factors [11,75,76]. In total, they can result in irreversible patient strain similar to scarring in bone disease and in lost opportunities with respect to personal, social, and professional life. Significant impairment may occur in patients with ineffective coping strategies and limited social support, even if they have a small burden. This impairment may be less in patients with effective coping strategies and strong social support networks, even if the burden is large.

Patients at risk for CLCI need to be identified by clinical, personal and psychosocial indicators and predictors of CLCI which need to be individually applied [18]. Among those factors, the following are to be considered:
1. clinical disease severity;
2. chronic course of disease;
3. early onset of psoriasis;
4. perception of stigmatization;
5. lack of social support;
6. negative impact on profession;
7. 'negative' mood/personality trait;
8. coping strategy;
9. quality of life;

10. behaviors putting the patient at risk; and
11. comorbidities.

Each of these factors requires accurate assessment either by clinical considerations or by specific tools. In particular, apart from any other single objectifiable risk factors, personality and social support of the patient can markedly affect the extent of CLCI and thus modulate the risks.

Conclusions for psoriasis management

The significant physical, psychological, social and economic burden, and stigmatization associated with psoriasis may result in an individual failing to achieve his 'full life potential'. Strategies currently recommended for the management of psoriasis tend to be highly technical in nature and regard people with the disease as a homogeneous population, with a similar clinical progression and a similar likelihood of treatment success. However, people with psoriasis represent a heterogeneous population with individual disease expressions and personal illness perceptions. A challenge to dermatological care is to realize long-lasting remittance of physical symptoms as well as a substantial improvement of quality of life. Therefore, the understanding of individual illness perceptions in patients with psoriasis is crucial when it comes to tailoring effective treatments with optimized outcomes. The immediate feedback of HRQoL measurements in the healthcare process could increase the therapeutic effectiveness as well as the cost-effectiveness of therapy when medical decisions are drawn earlier and closer to patient needs. In that sense, inclusion of HRQoL in the routine decision process favors individualized medicine in its best sense.

However, the complex association between these physical and psychological factors and QoL in this patient group is insufficiently investigated and not fully understood. There is broad agreement that Dermatologists, General Practitioners, and other healthcare professionals (HCPs) should routinely check the psychological and physical impact of psoriasis on people's lives when assessing the condition, according to latest guidance. In consultations between patients and their healthcare providers, several elements become crucial when it comes to providing adequate and comprehensive healthcare and addressing the relevant aspects of the disease [76–78]:

1. Exploration of a person's understanding of psoriasis and personal experiences with the disease in daily life.
2. Identification of personal, social, cultural, and physical issues contributing to the patient's QoL.
3. Acknowledgement of social and emotional consequences, particularly the distress that may be experienced in relation to personal social interactions with society.
4. Support in the development of coping strategies.

HCPs should address a virtual checklist, taking the relevant aspects of HRQoL of psoriasis patients into consideration with the aim that they incorporate the findings in a treatment strategy:

1. Try to find out if the patient has an increased burden due to perceived stigmatization.
2. Check patients' emotional status and the extent of 'positive' thinking and coping.
3. Discuss the coping profile of the patient and her/his personal beliefs in healing, her/his fears and the way she/he deals with the chronic disorder. Check also for personal resources and control attributions.
4. Explore the degree of social support and the patient's satisfaction with social relationships as a potential risk factor. It is well known that diseases of any severity and duration can be better tolerated and coped with when there is social support on the part of the family, friends, or others who are caring for the patient. Moreover, social support and social comfort are associated with better HRQoL. Therefore, lack of social/family/partner support and social isolation should be a warning sign for the dermatologist. In conclusion, explore the degree of social support and the patient's satisfaction with social relationships as a potential risk factor.
5. Find out whether the patient's professional opportunities have been met in full or whether they are at risk of being missed due to psoriasis.
6. Check for lifetime clinical severity and historical peak activity.

7. Include chronic course of disease as a potential CLCI factor.
8. Be specifically aware of CLCI factors in young psoriasis patients.
9. Risk behavior potentially inducing psoriasis should be included in any screening for CLCI risks.
10. Include QoL measurement and improvement in the management strategy of psoriasis. In addition to clinical outcomes, valid measures of QoL like the DLQI or the Skindex-29 or Skindex-17 should be routinely used for defining treatment goals in practice. Also, more recent assessment tools for the burden imposed on patients like the Psodisk may be applied.

There are already several reasons to recommend screening psoriasis patients for comorbidities. One more reason is the impact of comorbidities on CLCI. Evidence-based recommendations for screening have been published and screening algorithms tools are in the process of development.

References

1   Russo PAJ, Ilchef R, Cooper AJ. Psychiatric morbidity in psoriasis: a review. *Australas J Dermatol*. 2004:45:155-161.

2   Nelson PA, Barker Z, Griffiths CEM, Cordingley L, Chew-Graham CA. 'On the surface': a qualitative study of GPs' and patients' perspectives on psoriasis. *BMC Fam Pract*. 2013;14:158.

3   Fortune DG, Richards HL, Main C, Griffiths CEM. What patients with psoriasis believe about their condition. *J Am Acad Dermatol*. 1998;39:196-201.

4   Jong EM de, Seegers BA, Gulinck MK, Boezeman JB, van de Kerkhof PC. Psoriasis of the nails associated with disability in a large number of patients: results of a recent interview with 1,728 patients. *Dermatology*. 1996;193:300-303.

5   Zachariae R, Zachariae H, Blomqvist K, et al. Quality of life in 6497 Nordic patients with psoriasis. *Br J Dermatol*. 2002;146:1006-1016.

6   Wahl AK, Robinson HS, Langeland E, Larsen MH, Krogstad A, Moum T. Clinical characteristics associated with illness perception in psoriasis. *Acta Derm Venereol*. 2014;94:271-275.

7   Gelfand JM, Feldman SR, Stern RS, Thomas J, Rolstad T, Margolis DJ. Determinants of quality of life in patients with psoriasis: a study from the US population. *J Am Acad Dermatol*. 2004;51:704-708.

8   Augustin M, Reich K, Glaeske G, Schaefer I, Radtke M. Co-morbidity and age-related prevalence of psoriasis: Analysis of health insurance data in Germany. *Acta Derm Venereol*. 2010;90:147-151.

9   Reich K. The concept of psoriasis as a systemic inflammation: implications for disease management. *J Eur Acad Dermatol Venereol*. 2012;26:3-11.

10   Montaudié H, Albert-Sabonnadière C, Acquacalda E, et al. Impact of systemic treatment of psoriasis on inflammatory parameters and markers of comorbidities and cardiovascular risk: results of a prospective longitudinal observational study. *J Eur Acad Dermatol Venereol*. 2014;28:1186-1191.

11   Kimball AB, Gieler U, Linder D, Sampogna F, Warren RB, Augustin M. Psoriasis: is the impairment to a patient's life cumulative? *J Eur Acad Dermatol Venereol*. 2010;24:989-1004.

12   Reich K, Mrowietz U. Treatment goals in psoriasis. *J Dtsch Dermatol Ges*. 2007;5:566-574.

13   Krueger G, Koo J, Lebwohl M, Menter A, Stern RS, Rolstad T. The impact of psoriasis on quality of life: results of a 1998 National Psoriasis Foundation patient-membership survey. *Arch Dermatol*. 2001;137:280-284.

14   Dubertret L, Mrowietz U, Ranki A, et al. European patient perspectives on the impact of psoriasis: the EUROPSO patient membership survey. *Br J Dermatol*. 2006;155:729-736.

15   Blome C, Simianer S, Purwins S, et al. Time needed for treatment is the major predictor of quality of life in psoriasis. *Dermatology*. 2010;221:154-159.

16   Kimball AB, Jacobson C, Weiss S, Vreeland MG, Wu Y. The psychosocial burden of psoriasis. *Am J Clin Dermatol*. 2005;6:383-392.

17   Fortune DG, Richards HL, Griffiths CEM, Main CJ. Psychological stress, distress and disability in patients with psoriasis: consensus and variation in the contribution of illness perceptions, coping and alexithymia. *Br J Clin Psychol*. 2002;41:157-174.

18   Augustin M. Cumulative life course impairment: identifying patients at risk. *Curr Probl Dermatol*. 2013;44:74-81.

19   Koo J. Population-based epidemiologic study of psoriasis with emphasis on quality of life assessment. *Dermatol Clin*. 1996;14:485-496.

20   Rapp SR, Feldman SR, Exum ML, Fleischer AB, Reboussin DM. Psoriasis causes as much disability as other major medical diseases. *J Am Acad Dermatol*. 1999;41:401-407.

21   Richards HL, Fortune DG, Weidmann A, Sweeney SKT, Griffiths CEM. Detection of psychological distress in patients with psoriasis: low consensus between dermatologist and patient. *Br J Dermatol*. 2004;151:1227-1233.

22   Ware JE, Sherbourne CD. The MOS 36-item short-form health survey (SF-36). I. Conceptual framework and item selection. *Med Care*. 1992;30:473-483.

23   McHorney CA, Ware JE, Raczek AE. The MOS 36-Item Short-Form Health Survey (SF-36): II. Psychometric and clinical tests of validity in measuring physical and mental health constructs. *Med Care*. 1993;31:247-263.

24   Rabin R, Charro F de. EQ-5D: a measure of health status from the EuroQol Group. *Ann Med*. 2001;33:337-343.

25   Finlay AY, Khan GK. Dermatology Life Quality Index (DLQI)–a simple practical measure for routine clinical use. *Clin Exp Dermatol*. 1994;19:210-216.

26   Augustin M, Zschocke I, Lange S, Seidenglanz K, Amon U. Lebensqualität bei Haut-erkrankungen: Vergleich verschiedener Lebensqualitäts-Fragebögen bei Psoriasis und atopischer Dermatitis. *Hautarzt*. 1999;50:715-722.

27   Finlay AY, Kelly SE. Psoriasis–an index of disability. *Clin Exp Dermatol*. 1987;12:8-11.

28   Lewis VJ, Finlay AY. Two decades experience of the Psoriasis Disability Index. *Dermatology*. 2005;210:261-268.

29   Augustin M, Krüger K, Radtke MA, Schwippl I, Reich K. Disease severity, quality of life and health care in plaque-type psoriasis: a multicenter cross-sectional study in Germany. *Dermatology*. 2008;216:366-372.

30   Nast A, Boehncke WH, Mrowietz U, et al. S3-Guidelines on the treatment of psoriasis vulgaris (English version). Update. *J Dtsch Dermatol Ges*. 2012;10:1-95.

31   Mrowietz U, Kragballe K, Reich K, et al. Definition of treatment goals for moderate to severe psoriasis: a European consensus. *Arch Dermatol Res*. 2011;303:1-10.

32   Radtke MA, Reich K, Blome C, Rustenbach S, Augustin M. Prevalence and clinical features of psoriatic arthritis and joint complaints in 2009 patients with psoriasis: results of a German national survey. *J Eur Acad Dermatol Venereol*. 2009;23:683-691.

33   Hongbo Y, Thomas CL, Harrison MA, Salek MS, Finlay AY. Translating the science of quality of life into practice: what do dermatology life quality index scores mean? *J Invest Dermatol*. 2005;125:659-664.

34 Hariram P, Mosam A, Aboobaker J, Esterhuizen T. Quality of life in psoriasis patients in KwaZulu Natal, South Africa. *Indian J Dermatol Venereol Leprol*. 2011;77:333-334.

35 Aghaei S, Moradi A, Ardekani GS. Impact of psoriasis on quality of life in Iran. *Indian J Dermatol Venereol Leprol*. 2009;75:220.

36 Lin T, See L, Shen Y, Liang C, Chang H, Lin Y. Quality of life in patients with psoriasis in northern Taiwan. *Chang Gung Med J*. 2011;34:186-196.

37 Gelfand JM, Feldman SR, Stern RS, Thomas J, Rolstad T, Margolis DJ. Determinants of quality of life in patients with psoriasis: a study from the US population. *J Am Acad Dermatol*. 2004;51:704-708.

38 Ginsburg IH, Link BG. Feelings of stigmatization in patients with psoriasis. *J Am Acad Dermatol*. 1989;20:53-63.

39 Richards HL, Fortune DG, Main CJ, Griffiths CEM. Stigmatization and psoriasis. *Br J Dermatol*. 2003;149:209-211.

40 Korte J de, Sprangers MA, Mombers FM, Bos JD. Quality of life in patients with psoriasis: a systematic literature review. *J Investig Dermatol Symp Proc*. 2004;9:140-147.

41 Gaikwad R, Deshpande S, Raje S, Dhamdhere DV, Ghate MR. Evaluation of functional impairment in psoriasis. *Indian J Dermatol Venereol Leprol*. 2006;72:37-40.

42 Graça Pereira M, Brito L, Smith T. Dyadic adjustment, family coping, body image, quality of life and psychological morbidity in patients with psoriasis and their partners. *Int J Behav Med*. 2012;19:260-269.

43 Eghlileb AM, Davies EEG, Finlay AY. Psoriasis has a major secondary impact on the lives of family members and partners. *Br J Dermatol*. 2007;156:1245-1250.

44 Picardi A, Abeni D, Renzi C, Braga M, Puddu P, Pasquini P. Increased psychiatric morbidity in female outpatients with skin lesions on visible parts of the body. *Acta Derm Venereol*. 2001;81:410-414.

45 Sojević Timotijević Z, Janković S, Trajković G, et al. Identification of psoriatic patients at risk of high quality of life impairment. *J Dermatolog Treat*. 2013;40:797-804.

46 Young M. The psychological and social burdens of psoriasis. *Dermatol Nurs*. 2005;17:15-19.

47 Varni JW, Globe DR, Gandra SR, Harrison DJ, Hooper M, Baumgartner S. Health-related quality of life of pediatric patients with moderate to severe plaque psoriasis: comparisons to four common chronic diseases. *Eur J Pediatr*. 2012;171:485-492.

48 Ayala F, Sampogna F, Romano G et al. The impact of psoriasis on work-related problems: a multicenter cross-sectional survey. *J Eur Acad Dermatol Venereol*. 2014;28:1623-1632.

49 Hughes JE, Barraclough BM, Hamblin LG, White JE. Pschiatric symptoms in dermatology patients. *Br J Psychol*. 1983;143:51-54.

50 Horn EJ, Fox KM, Patel V, Chiou C, Dann F, Lebwohl M. Association of patient-reported psoriasis severity with income and employment. *J Am Acad Dermatol*. 2007;57:963-971.

51 Fowler JF, Duh MS, Rovba L, et al. The impact of psoriasis on health care costs and patient work loss. *J Am Acad Dermatol*. 2008;59:772-780.

52 Kimball AB, Yu AP, Signorovitch J et al. The effects of adalimumab treatment and psoriasis severity on self-reported work productivity and activity impairment for patients with moderate to severe psoriasis. *J Am Acad Dermatol*. 2012;66:e67-e76.

53 Pearce DJ, Singh S, Balkrishnan R, Kulkarni A, Fleischer AB, Feldman SR. The negative impact of psoriasis on the workplace. *J Dermatolog Treat*. 2006;17;24-28.

54 Reich K, Schenkel B, Zhao N, et al. Ustekinumab decreases work limitations, improves work productivity, and reduces work days missed in patients with moderate-to-severe psoriasis: results from PHOENIX 2. *J Dermatolog Treat*. 2011;22:337-347.

55 Chan B, Hales B, Shear N, et al. Work-related lost productivity and its economic impact on Canadian patients with moderate to severe psoriasis. *J Cutan Med Surg*. 2009;13:192-197.

56 Feldman SR, Fleischer AB, Reboussin DM, et al. The economic impact of psoriasis increases with psoriasis severity. *J Am Acad Dermatol*. 1997;37:564-569.

57 Kotsis K, Voulgari PV, Tsifetaki N et al. Anxiety and depressive symptoms and illness perceptions in psoriatic arthritis and associations with physical health-related quality of life. *Arthritis Care Res (Hoboken)*. 2012;64:1593-1601.

58 Augustin M, Holland B, Dartsch D, Langenbruch A, Radtke MA. Adherence in the treatment of psoriasis: a systematic review. *Dermatology*. 2011;222:363-374.

59 Richards HL, Fortune DG, Griffiths CEM. Adherence to treatment in patients with psoriasis. *J Eur Acad Dermatol Venereol*. 2006;20:370-379.

60 Kimball AB, Gladman D, Gelfand JM, et al. National Psoriasis Foundation clinical consensus on psoriasis comorbidities and recommendations for screening. *J Am Acad Dermatol*. 2008;58:1031-1042.

61 Daudén E, Castañeda S, Suárez C, et al. Clinical practice guideline for an integrated approach to comorbidity in patients with psoriasis. *J Eur Acad Dermatol Venereol*. 2013;27:1387-1404.

62 Ljosaa TM, Rustoen T, Mörk C, et al. Skin pain and discomfort in psoriasis: an exploratory study of symptom prevalence and characteristics. *Acta Derm. Venereol*. 2010;90:39-45.

63 McKenna KE, Stern RS. The impact of psoriasis on the quality of life of patients from the 16-center PUVA follow-up cohort. *J Am Acad Dermatol*. 1997;36:388-394.

64 Sampogna F, Gisondi P, Melchi CF, Amerio P, Girolomoni G, Abeni D. Prevalence of symptoms experienced by patients with different clinical types of psoriasis. *Br J Dermatol*. 2004;151:594-599.

65 Yosipovitch G, Goon A, Wee J, Chan YH, Goh CL. The prevalence and clinical characteristics of pruritus among patients with extensive psoriasis. *Br J Dermatol*. 2000;143:969-973.

66 Amatya B, Wennersten G, Nordlind K. Patients' perspective of pruritus in chronic plaque psoriasis: a questionnaire-based study. *J Eur Acad Dermatol Venereol*. 2008;22:822-826.

67 Globe D, Bayliss MS, Harrison DJ. The impact of itch symptoms in psoriasis: results from physician interviews and patient focus groups. *Health Qual Life Outcomes*. 2009;7:62.

68 Choi J, Koo JYM. Quality of life issues in psoriasis. *J Am Acad Dermatol*. 2003;49:S57-S61.

69 Zachariae R, Zachariae C, Ibsen HHW, Mortensen JT, Wulf HC. Psychological symptoms and quality of life of dermatology outpatients and hospitalized dermatology patients. *Acta Derm Venereol*. 2004;84:205-212.

70 Wahl A, Moum T, Hanestad BR, Wiklund I. The relationship between demographic and clinical variables, and quality of life aspects in patients with psoriasis. *Qual Life Res*. 1999;8:319-326.

71 Ljosaa TM, Mork C, Stubhaug A, Moum T, Wahl AK. Skin pain and skin discomfort is associated with quality of life in patients with psoriasis. *J Eur Acad Dermatol Venereol*. 2012;26:29-35.

72 Feuerhahn J, Blome C, Radtke MA, Augustin M. Validation of the patient benefit index for the assessment of patient-relevant benefit in the treatment of psoriasis. *Arch Dermatol Res*. 2012;304:433-441.

73 Blome C, Augustin M, Behechtnejad J, Rustenbach SJ. Dimensions of patient needs in dermatology: subscales of the patient benefit index. *Arch Dermatol Res*. 2011;303:11-17.

74 Krenzer S, Radtke M, Schmitt-Rau K, Augustin M. Characterization of patient-reported outcomes (pro) in moderate to severe psoriasis. *Dermatology*. 2011;223:80-86.

75 Bhatti ZU, Salek MS, Finlay AY. Major life changing decisions and cumulative life course impairment. *J Eur Acad Dermatol Venereol*. 2011;25:245-246.

76 Augustin M, Alvaro-Gracia JM, Bagot M, et al. A framework for improving the quality of care for people with psoriasis. *J Eur Acad Dermatol Venereol*. 2012;26:1-16.

77 Mrowietz U, Kragballe K, Nast A, Reich K. Strategies for improving the quality of care in psoriasis with the use of treatment goals--a report on an implementation meeting. *J Eur Acad Dermatol Venereol*. 2011;25:1-13.

78 Jankowiak B, Sekmistrz S, Kowalewska B, Niczyporuk W, Krajewska-Kułak E. Satisfaction with life in a group of psoriasis patients. *Postepy Dermatol Alergol*. 2013;30:85-90.

CPSIA information can be obtained
at www.ICGtesting.com
Printed in the USA
LVOW02s2337100516
487559LV00009BA/38/P